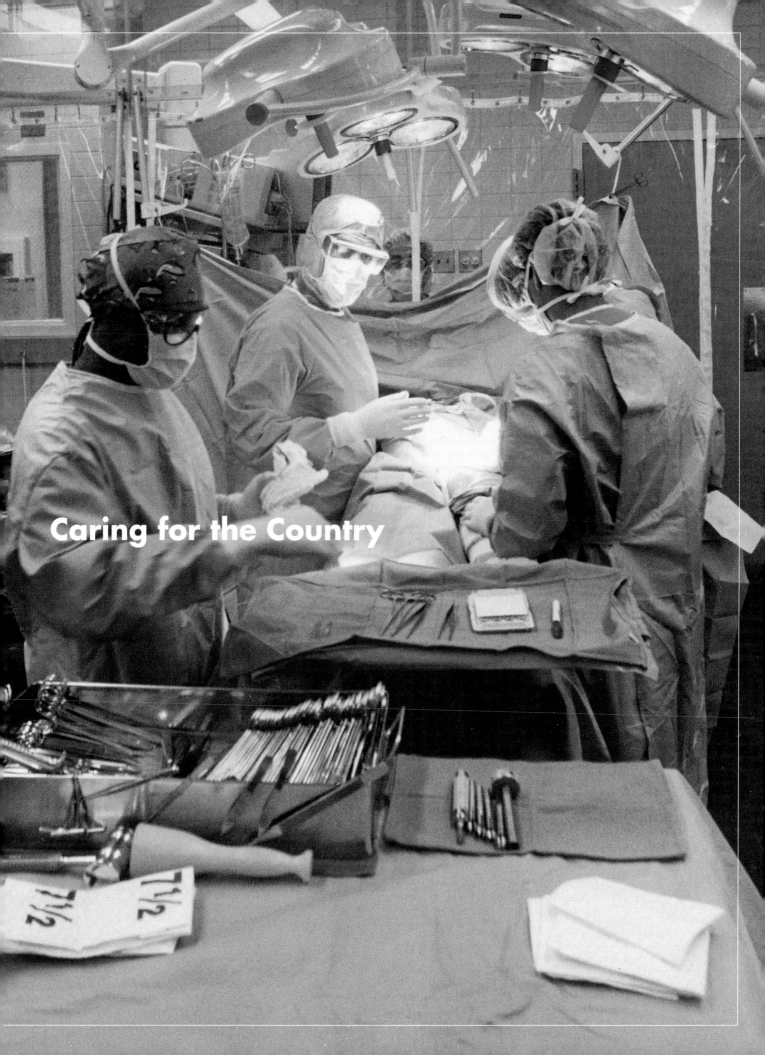

Caring for the Country

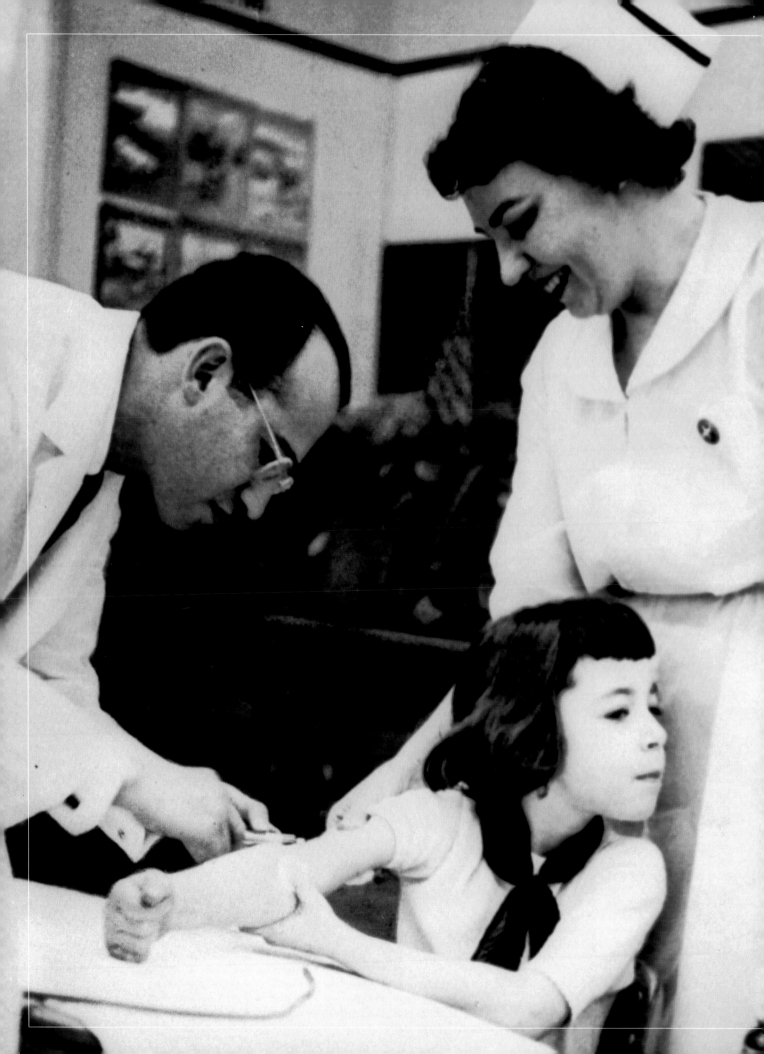

Caring for the Country

**A History and Celebration
of the First 150 Years
of the American Medical Association**

American Medical Association
Chicago

© 1997 by the American Medical Association

For illustration credits, please see page 174.

Printed in the USA.
All rights reserved.

Additional copies of this book (Product Number OP047697)
may be ordered by calling, toll free: 800 621-8335.

Internet address: http://www.ama-assn.org

ISBN: 0-89970-840-4

AF58:96-259:15M:2/97

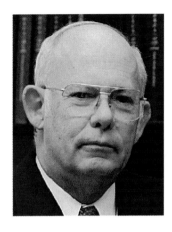

Preface

The American Medical Association celebrates its 150th anniversary by rededicating ourselves and our members to our historic mission of caring for the country while leading the medical profession toward the next century.

We possess a rich and noble heritage that began in 1847 when Nathan Davis, MD, and his colleagues founded the AMA to "promote the science and art of medicine and the betterment of public health."

This book tells the story of America's best medicine, a story inspired by the hope, hard work, and triumph of hundreds of thousands of dedicated men and women who followed Dr Davis as AMA members.

While much has changed in the past century and a half, a bedrock of basic principles still forms the AMA's foundation, principles such as patient advocacy, ethics, education, professionalism, standard setting, and quality of care. These principles are so lastingly fundamental to the physician's calling that they transcend the passage of time and generations. By changing with the times without surrendering these firmly rooted values, the AMA has earned the stature of a true American presence.

We are an original American icon, more a national institution than a national organization, respected as a leader, trusted as the protector of the patient-physician relationship, and relied on as the voice of medicine — past, present, and future.

The reason we are so respected by the public and patients we serve is because our physicians believe that AMA membership is:

- **A pledge that AMA members always put the interests of their patients first.**

- **A promise that the AMA Code of Medical Ethics guides the AMA physician.**

- **A personal statement that the AMA physician is dedicated to the good health of both patients and the medical profession.**

That is our memorial to the AMA members of the past and our legacy to the AMA members of the future. And this is why the AMA — at 150 years of age — is America's brightest and best medicine for the new millennium.

P. John Seward, MD, Executive Vice President
American Medical Association
Chicago, Ill, 1997

Acknowledgments

The American Medical Association wishes to thank the following:

Lewis Crampton
Vice President, Communications
Chair of 150th Anniversary Committee and Executive Editor

Dick Walt
Editor, *American Medical News*, 1983 to 1991
Writer

Patricia Dragisic
Managing Editor, Trade Publishing
Project Manager

Allen J. Podraza
Manager, Records Management and Archives
Illustrations Editor

Thanks for their many contributions also to the following: M. Frances Dyra, AMA Product Line Management; Roberta Gilmore, AMA Office Services, for editorial assistance; Ted Grudzinski, AMA Photography, for shooting new pictures for the book; Hafeman Design Group Inc, Chicago, for the book design; Robert Hobart, Vice President, AMA Corporate Services; Larry Jellen, Vice President, AMA Marketing; Jane Kenamore, AMA Records Management and Archives, for her dedicated research on the illustrations and timelines; George Kruto, Chicago, for the index; Katherine A. Landeck, AMA Corporate Law; Cynthia Leverett, AMA Communications, for administrative assistance; Nicole Netter, Lake Bluff, Ill, for copyediting; Rosalyn Robinson, AMA Marketing Services, for coordinating all phases of production; Ross Rubin, Vice President, AMA Legislative Activities; Tim Ryan, AMA Marketing, marketing manager; Debra A. Smith, AMA Trade Publishing, for administrative support; Rhonda Taira, AMA Marketing Services; Robert Williamson, AMA Records Management and Archives, for his enthusiastic assistance on photo research; and Roxanne Young, *JAMA*.

Special thanks to the AMA Board of Trustees (see facing page), 1996–1997, for planning the big birthday celebration!

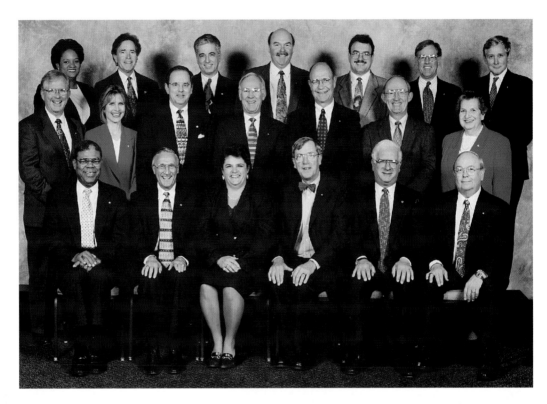

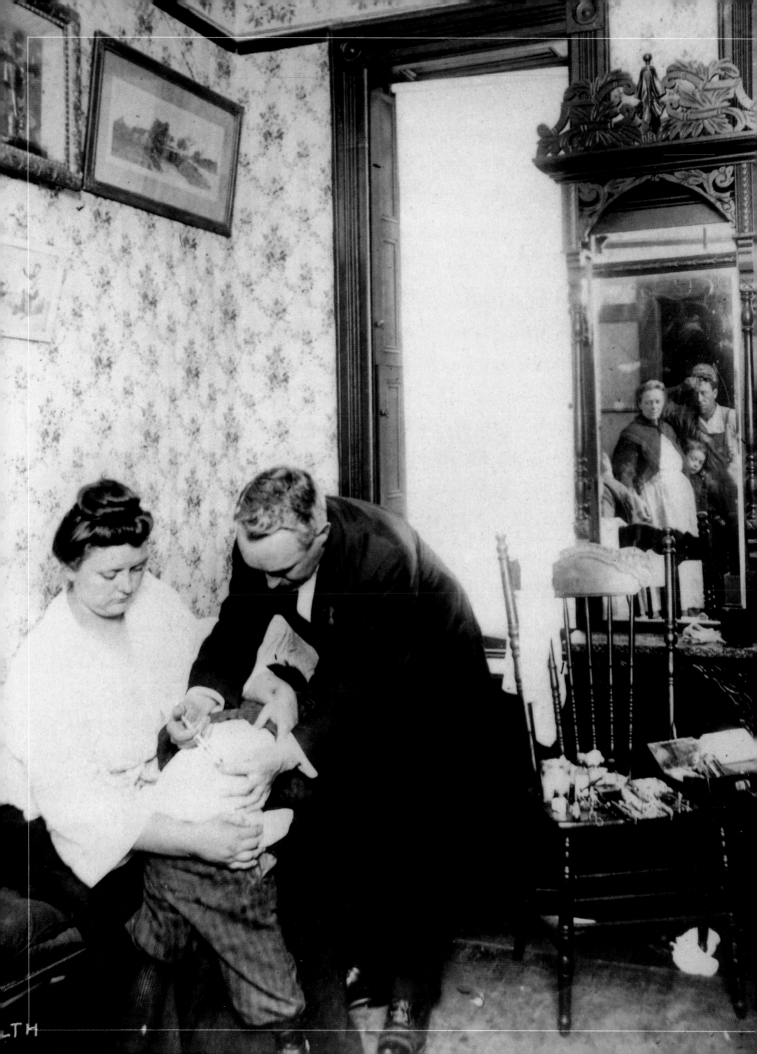

Table of Contents

Highlights in AMA History

1847

Founding of AMA at Academy of Natural Sciences in Philadelphia (Founder Nathan Davis)

AMA Committee on Medical Education appointed

AMA Code of Medical Ethics written and published

AMA establishes standards for preliminary medical education and for the degree of MD

1848

AMA recommends that the value of anesthetic agents in medicine, surgery, and obstetrics be determined

1849

AMA establishes a board to analyze quack remedies and nostrums and to enlighten the public in regard to the nature and danger of such remedies

1858

AMA establishes Committee on Ethics

1873

AMA Judicial Council founded to deal with ethical and constitutional issues

1883

Journal of the American Medical Association founded; Nathan Davis is first editor

US and World Events

Cholera epidemic in US kills people living in inner cities and on the trail to the California Gold Rush

1849

Civil War

1861 • 1865

Thomas Edison invents electric light bulb

1879

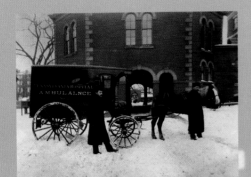

1910

The Flexner Report, *Medical Education in the United States and Canada,* funded by the Carnegie Foundation and supported by the AMA, is published and facilitates new standards for medical schools. The report exposes many diploma mills

1899

AMA urges local boards of health to require smallpox vaccination

1912

The Federation of State Medical Boards is established, accepting AMA's rating of medical schools as authoritative

1898

AMA Committee on Scientific Research is established to provide grants for fostering medical research

1906 • 1907

AMA Council on Medical Education inspects 160 medical schools and classifies them into three groups: A = acceptable; B = doubtful; and C = unacceptable

1901

AMA reorganizes, creating the House of Delegates

Pure Food and Drug Act passes

HMS *Titanic* goes down with 1513 lives lost

Wilhelm Roentgen discovers x-rays

1906

Orville and Wilbur Wright make first successful airplane flight

1894

1912

1903

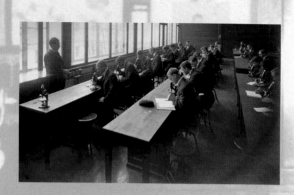

1914

AMA Council on Medical Education sets standards for hospital internship programs and publishes first list of approved hospitals offering such programs

1923

AMA adopts standards for medical specialty training

1922

Woman's Auxiliary to the AMA is organized to assist the AMA in the advancement of medicine and public health

1913

AMA establishes a department to gather and disseminate information concerning health fraud and quackery

1924

Morris Fishbein begins 25-year tenure as editor of *JAMA* and *Hygeia*

World War I

1914
•
1918

Influenza pandemic kills more people worldwide than died during World War I

1918
•
1919

1927

AMA Council on Medical Education and Hospitals publishes first list of hospitals approved for residency training

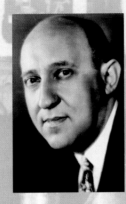

1937

AMA asks county medical societies to share the burden of caring for poor patients

1934

Official recognition of medical specialty boards begins through collaborative efforts of the AMA Council on Medical Education and the Advisory Board for Medical Specialties (and later by its successor, the American Board of Medical Specialties)

1942

The AMA Council on Medical Education and the Association of American Medical Colleges establish the Liaison Committee on Medical Education to accredit programs leading to the MD degree

1943

AMA opens office in Washington, DC

1951

Joint Commission on Accreditation of Hospitals is formed by AMA, the American College of Surgeons, American College of Physicians, American Hospital Association, and Canadian Medical Association

AMA Education and Research Foundation established to help medical schools meet expenses and to help medical students

Gaston Leon Ramon develops active immunization against tetanus (and later diphtheria)

1927

Alexander Fleming discovers penicillin

1928

World War II

**1939
•
1945**

Improvements in trauma surgery during Korean Conflict

**1950
•
1953**

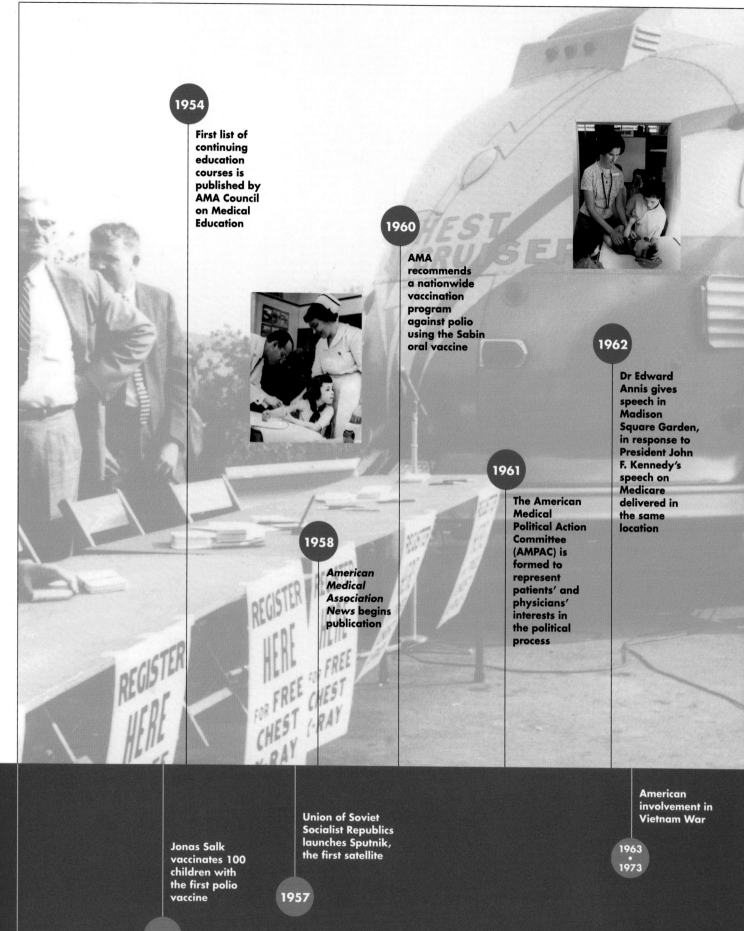

1954

First list of continuing education courses is published by AMA Council on Medical Education

1960

AMA recommends a nationwide vaccination program against polio using the Sabin oral vaccine

1962

Dr Edward Annis gives speech in Madison Square Garden, in response to President John F. Kennedy's speech on Medicare delivered in the same location

1961

The American Medical Political Action Committee (AMPAC) is formed to represent patients' and physicians' interests in the political process

1958

American Medical Association News begins publication

American involvement in Vietnam War

Union of Soviet Socialist Republics launches Sputnik, the first satellite

Jonas Salk vaccinates 100 children with the first polio vaccine

1963
•
1973

1957

1952

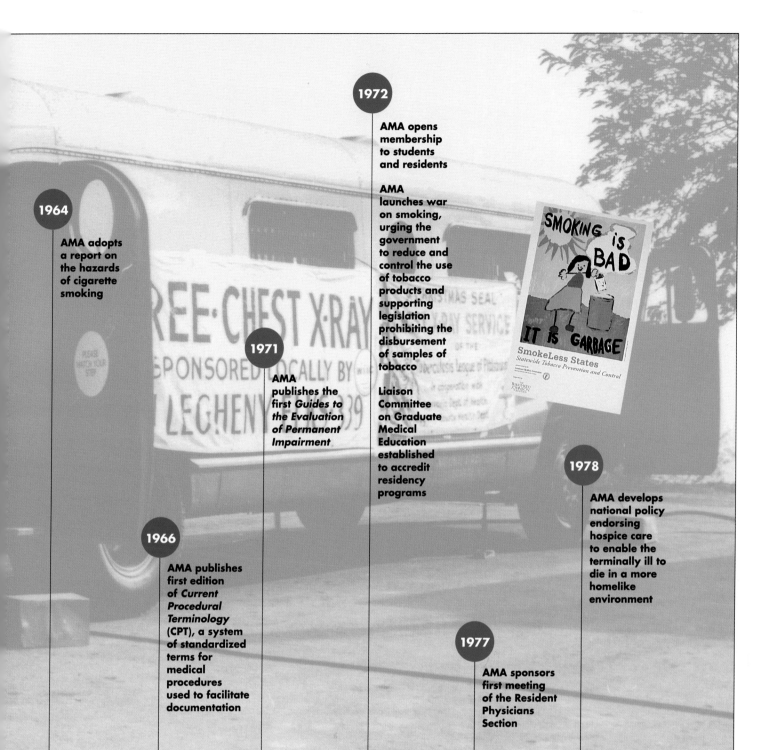

1964

AMA adopts a report on the hazards of cigarette smoking

1971

AMA publishes the first *Guides to the Evaluation of Permanent Impairment*

1966

AMA publishes first edition of *Current Procedural Terminology* (CPT), a system of standardized terms for medical procedures used to facilitate documentation

1972

AMA opens membership to students and residents

AMA launches war on smoking, urging the government to reduce and control the use of tobacco products and supporting legislation prohibiting the disbursement of samples of tobacco

Liaison Committee on Graduate Medical Education established to accredit residency programs

1978

AMA develops national policy endorsing hospice care to enable the terminally ill to die in a more homelike environment

1977

AMA sponsors first meeting of the Resident Physicians Section

1965

US Congress passes bill authorizing Medicare and Medicaid

1967

Christian Barnard of South Africa transplants first human heart

1976

United States celebrates its bicentennial

1979

Global Commission for the Certification of Smallpox Eradication officially announces demise of the disease

SMOKING is BAD IT IS GARBAGE

SmokeLess States
Statewide Tobacco Prevention and Control

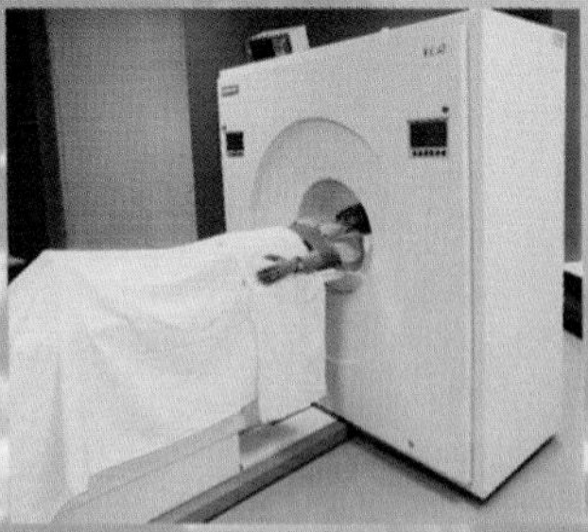

1983

AMA urges a smoke-free society by the year 2000

Hospital Medical Staff Section, now the Organized Medical Staff Section, is established within the AMA

1989

AMA develops National HIV Policy reiterating physicians' ethical responsibilities to treat HIV patients whose condition is within the physicians' realm of competence

1986

AMA passes resolution opposing acts of discrimination against AIDS patients and any legislation that would lead to such categorical discrimination or that would affect patient-physician confidentiality

1982

George Lundberg begins serving as editor-in-chief of *JAMA* and Scientific Publications

AMA Consumer Publishing program begins with the *AMA Family Medical Guide*, published by Random House

1990

AMA moves into new building at 515 N State St, Chicago

AMA adopts guidelines governing gifts to physicians from the pharmaceutical industry

Berlin Wall comes down

1989

Sandra Day O'Connor is the first woman appointed to US Supreme Court

Scientists discover the virus that causes AIDS

1981

1984

1995

AMA launches grassroots campaign for professional liability reform

AMA drafts the Patient Protection Act II bill to protect patients through a proposed ban on gag clauses and other practices of insurance plans that infringe on the physician-patient relationship

AMA launches its Website on the Internet, featuring highlights of *JAMA*, the specialty journals, *American Medical News*, and other AMA news of interest

1993

AMA passes resolution declaring that physician-assisted suicide is fundamentally inconsistent with the physician's professional role

1991

AMA proposes reform of the US health care system (Health Access America) to include expansion of health insurance coverage

AMA launches campaign against family violence

1992

AMA calls on tobacco companies to refrain from engaging in advertising practices that target children

1996

AMA scores crucial victories in Washington for physicians and patients with legislation on antitrust relief, health insurance reform, and restriction of tobacco sales to childen

1997

AMA celebrates sesquicentennial of its founding

1991

Persian Gulf War

1993

Israel Prime Minister Yitzhak Rabin and Palestinian leader Yasser Arafat sign Israeli-Palestinian peace accords in Washington, DC

JAMA
July 28/26, 1992
The Journal of the American Medical Association

Netscape: Official American Medical Association (AMA) Home Page

American Medical Association

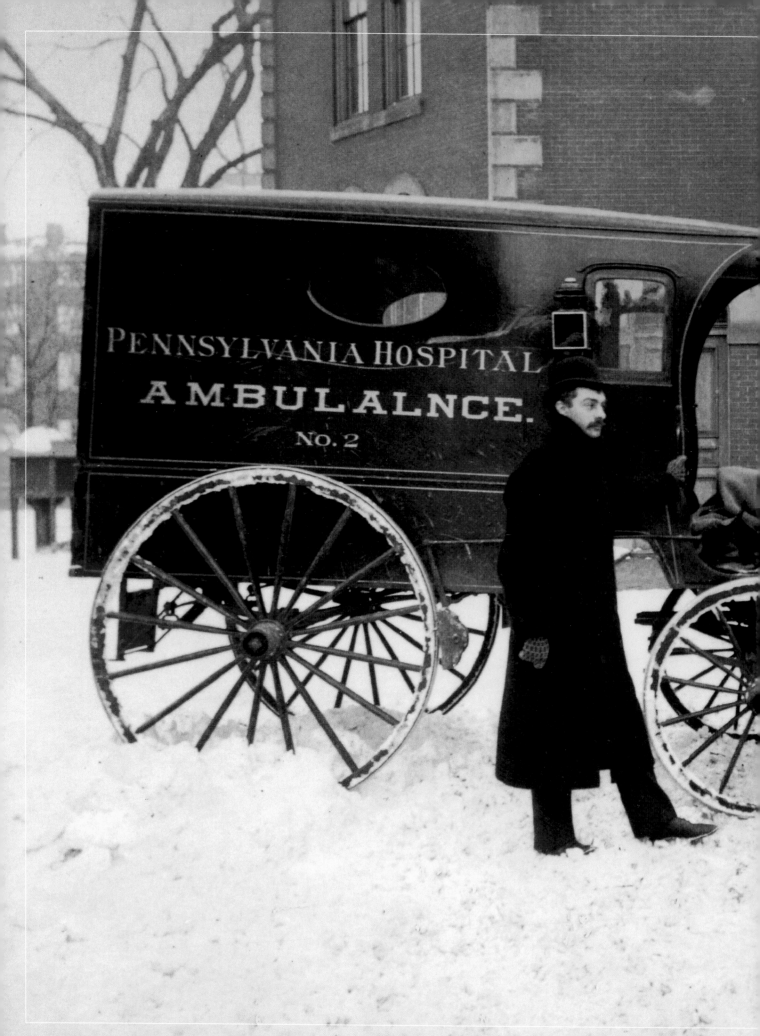

As Dr Davis was writing his now-historic document, James K. Polk was about to succeed John Tyler as president of the United States (there were 28 states then). Ether anesthesia was a year old. The first telegraph message had been sent only a year before, from Baltimore to Washington, DC. Oberlin College in Ohio had just become the first college to confer degrees on women.

While there was no national association of physicians, state medical societies existed in many areas. The first was the New Jersey State Medical Society, launched in 1766. Before the AMA was founded, state societies had been formed in a dozen more states and in numerous metropolitan counties. The *New England Journal of Medicine* had begun publication in 1820.

Thus, the call to form a national organization came at a propitious time, and Dr Davis proved to be the right man for the right job at the right time. When his resolution was adopted in 1845, Dr Davis was named chairman of a committee to organize the first National Convention. He devoted much of the next several months to efforts to promote the meeting among medical organizations and medical schools.

On May 5, 1846, about 80 representatives of medical societies and colleges in 16 different states convened at New York University. After some preliminary parliamentary skirmishing, Dr Davis was named to chair a committee to develop a policy statement to be considered at the next meeting. On the following day, Dr Davis' committee presented four proposals:

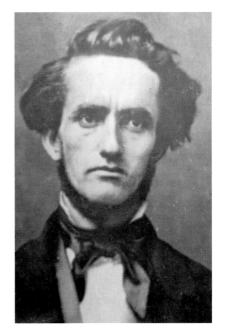

Nathan S. Davis, MD: his role in founding the AMA was followed by 4 decades of service.

- **First, That it is expedient for the medical profession of the United States to institute a National Medical Association.**

- **Secondly, That it is desirable that a uniform and elevated standard of requirements for the degree of M.D. should be adopted by all the medical schools in the United States.**

- **Thirdly, That it is desirable that young men, before being received as students of medicine, should have acquired a suitable preliminary education.**

- **Fourthly, That it is expedient that the medical profession in the United States should be governed by the same code of medical ethics.**

Dr Davis' committee also recommended appointment of a committee to plan the founding meeting of the new organization, to be held in Philadelphia in May 1847.

The beginnings of the AMA went largely unnoticed in the press of national events that year — most notably, the war between the United States and Mexico. As a result of that conflict, the United States would obtain the land that would become Texas, California, Arizona, New Mexico, Nevada, Utah, and part of Colorado. A treaty with Great Britain in the same year gave the United States the Oregon Territory to the 49th parallel, and Henry David Thoreau was jailed for tax resistance. The California gold rush was still 3 years away.

On May 5, 1847, about 250 delegates met at the Academy of Natural Sciences in Philadelphia and formed the American Medical Association. The delegates were from 40 medical societies and 28 medical schools; in all, 28 of the 29 states then in the Union were represented. May 7, 1847, is the official birthday of the American Medical Association, the day that a resolution was passed to found the organization.

The AMA's constitution and first policies

One of the most important organizational policies — and one for which Dr Davis argued eloquently — was that the AMA would be an organization of state, county, and local medical societies and institutions and of medical colleges, rather than an organization of individuals elected by the society itself, as was common in professional organizations of that time.

H. Hayes Agnew, MD (white hair), performs leg surgery using ether anesthesia before an 1886 class of University of Pennsylvania medical students.

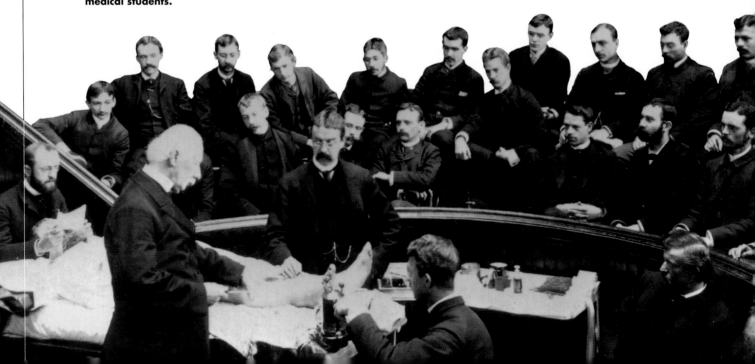

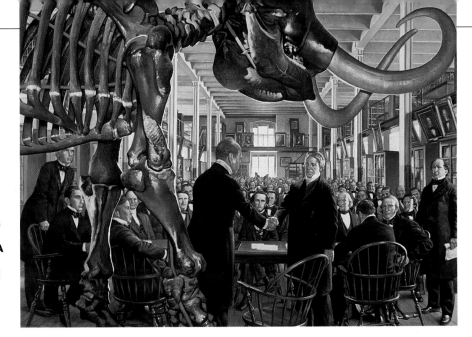

This painting depicts the May 7, 1847, founding of the AMA at Philadelphia's Academy of Natural Sciences. AMA President Nathaniel Chapman, MD, is in the foreground.

Another important step was the adoption of a series of resolutions regarding the prerequisites for the study of medicine and requiring a physician preceptor for each entering medical student; subsequent resolutions would address the length of the curriculum, minimum standards for training (including 3 months devoted to dissection), and a session of hospital practice — the forerunner of the internship.

Within 2 days of its formation, the AMA launched what became a ceaseless war on quackery, warning of the hazards of universal traffic in "secret" medicines. The first nationwide code of medical ethics was also introduced — several state societies had established different versions — drawing in large measure from the writings of Thomas Percival, the British ethicist who published the first major manuscript on medical ethics in 1803.

The first constitution set forth the principle of representation by delegates from medical societies and institutions, and the founders urged the formation of state and local associations. At the same time, committees were established on medical sciences, practical medicine, surgery, obstetrics, medical education, medical literature, and publication.

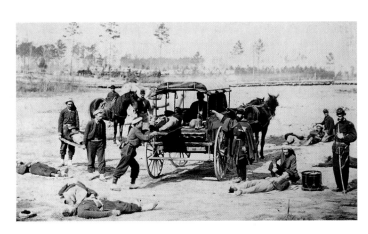

Wounded soldiers in the Civil War are treated on the battlefield.

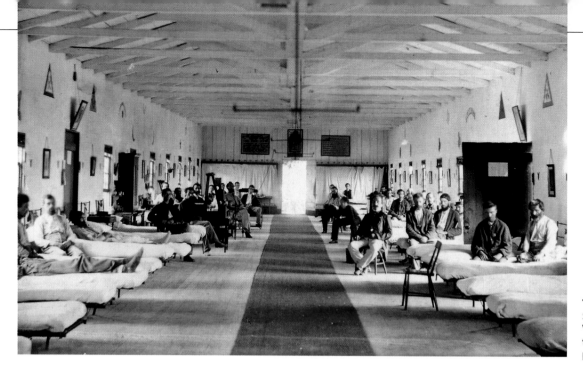

The Armory Square Hospital, Washington, DC, treated Civil War patients in 1864.

The first president was Nathaniel Chapman, MD, of Pennsylvania. Dr Chapman's words at the opening session of the 1848 meeting bear repeating, to help recall the founders' goals:

"The profession to which we belong, once venerated on account of its antiquity — its various and profound science — its elegant literature — its polite accomplishments — its virtues — has become corrupt and degenerate to the forfeiture of its social position and, with it, of the homage it formerly received spontaneously and universally."

In 1848, dues were established at $3 a year; delegates to the meeting asked the Board of Trustees to initiate a drive for new members.

The definitive history of the AMA's early years was published in 1947 by Morris Fishbein, MD, the long-time editor of *JAMA*. His detailed accounts of the AMA's early meetings — obviously based on close study of the proceedings — point out that in the early years of the Association, most of the time at the meetings was spent on reports on scientific progress. However, he occasionally noted developments that seem timely in today's environment.

In 1849, for example, a resolution urged physicians to present lectures "to enlighten the public mind in regard to the duties and responsibilities of the medical profession and their just claims to the confidence of the public." At the same meeting, Dr Fishbein noted, even though the AMA was only 2 years old, "many members were beginning to get a little weary of the length of time required to read the annual reports."

Also in 1849, the Committee on Medical Education provided a survey of medical education in Europe and compared it with the curriculum in each school in the United States.

In 1852 the AMA took one of its first looks at an international health problem, noting that in the stream of immigrants from Europe to the United States, many were transported in steerage, in appalling sanitary conditions, and without access to any form of medical care.

Public relations — not by that name — surfaced again in 1855, when a resolution urged that "reporters of the public press" be given every courtesy "to enable them to furnish full and accurate reports of the transactions."

In its first half-century,
education, ethics, and science
were AMA's chief concerns.

However, the early years of the AMA were preoccupied with the issues of education, ethics, and scientific advancements. Although the Civil War was imminent and there was turmoil across the nation, there is no indication that the Association considered this an issue for the medical profession, and there was no action addressing military preparedness.

The 1860s and the Civil War

The Civil War did force cancellation of AMA's meetings in 1861 and 1862. The meetings resumed in 1863, with Dr Davis serving as chairman of the Committee on Arrangements. At the 1864 meeting in New York, he was elected president of the AMA.

In his 1865 presidential address, Dr Davis voiced his gratification that the United States were again united, and described President Lincoln's assassination as "the climax of human wickedness." Dr Davis' concentration never strayed far from the AMA activities, however, and he expressed great disappointment that the Association's social schedule and crowded agenda precluded proper consideration of some of the more significant activities. A lifelong supporter of the temperance movement, he warned that "the attempt to eliminate from the program the entertainments has resulted only in exchanging one magnificent public banquet occupying one evening for three or four private ones during the annual session of the Association."

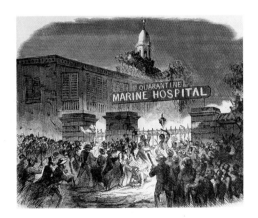

Rioters attacked a quarantine hospital for releasing patients during an 1858 yellow fever epidemic.

During the postwar period of reconstruction, the AMA made a concentrated effort to achieve rapprochement with the South. A Southerner, William O. Baldwin, MD, of Alabama, was elected president in 1868, and the annual convention was held in New Orleans in 1869. At that meeting, Dr Baldwin also spoke for reunification:

"At a time when every other organization has been shaken to its center by the passions of the deadliest hate; at a time when the most matured conservatism has been overmastered by the vindictive fury which has swayed the popular mind; you have been drawn hither from homes far distant over highways full of painful historic incidents, through territories watered by the blood and tears of a sorrowing nation, and you have assembled here as brothers and friends to unite your offerings to a common science."

It also was in the 1860s that the AMA took its first major look at specialization. Some physicians at the 1869 meeting warned that specialists "operate unfairly toward the general practitioner, in implying that he is incompetent to properly treat certain classes of disease, and narrowing his field of practice." However, the report went on to say, "It is natural that in any changes from old-beaten paths, there should be some temporary confusion, but…as soon as the relations between special and general practice become better adjusted…great advantages will accrue, even to the general practitioner."

The report also called on specialists and generalists alike to abide by the same rules of "etiquette" and stated, "It shall not be proper for specialists publicly to advertise themselves as such, or to assume any title not specially granted by a regular chartered college."

These actions did not resolve the issue, of course, and conflict continued for decades. Medical historian Lester King, MD, writing in the AMA's *Healthcare Resource and Reference Guide* in 1992, noted, "Medical practice had always involved competition for patients. The growth of specialism in the last third of the 19th century rendered the process more acute than ever. The struggle, however, was taking place in a constantly shifting environment. The entire culture was in flux, and the relation of physicians to each other and to their patients had to undergo severe and constant readjustments as the cultural and economic environment changed."

As the internal political struggles continued, however, the American Medical Association was slowly gaining in stature in the eyes of physicians and of the public. A measure of the esteem the organization had attained is found in the list of distinguished physicians who ascended to its presidency.

Facing page: Participants in AMA's 1889 meeting pose in Newport, RI.

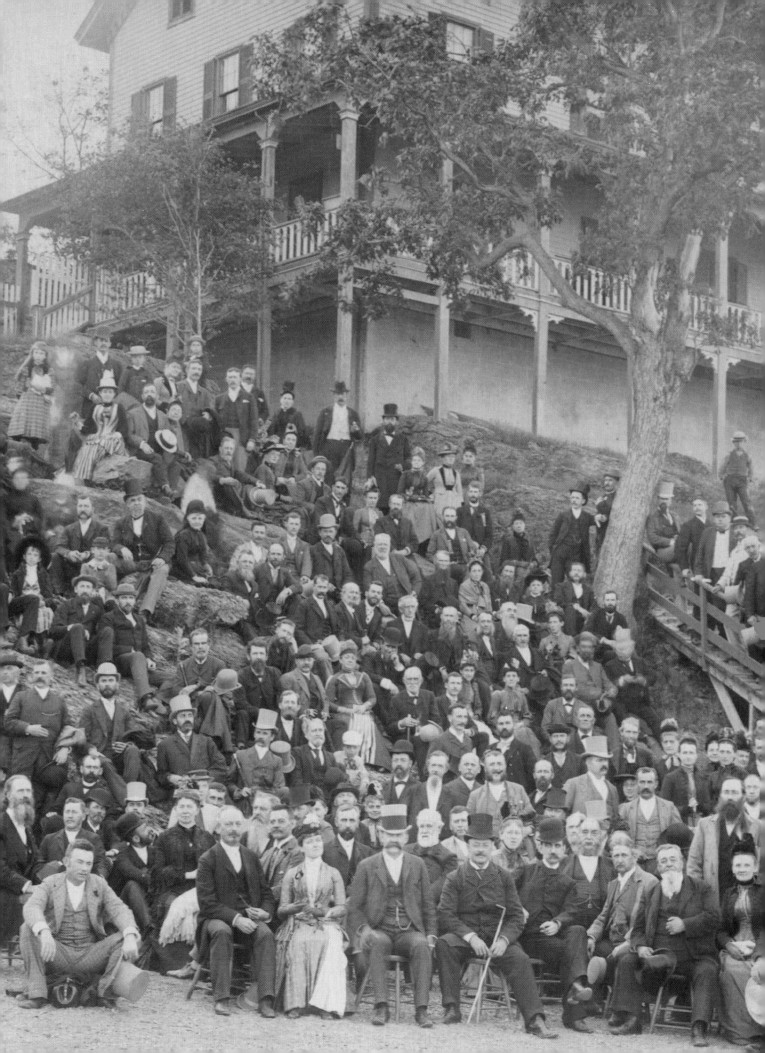

A historic issue: this is the first cover of the *Journal of the American Medical Association* (JAMA), July 14, 1883. Dr Nathan Davis was the first editor.

The first president, Nathaniel Chapman, MD, elected in 1847, had published *Elements of Therapeutics and Materia Medica* 30 years earlier, which went through seven editions. In 1820 he became the first editor of the *American Journal of Medical Sciences*.

In 1849, the AMA's president was John C. Warren, MD. It was in his surgical clinic in Boston in 1846 that ether was first used as an anesthetic. He was reported to have said at the time, "Gentlemen, this is no humbug."

George B. Wood, MD, the AMA's president in 1855, had been coauthor of the *United States Dispensatory* a decade earlier; he also published *Wood's Practice of Medicine* — hailed as the most important work on the subject at that time — in 1847.

The first textbook on obstetrics had been published by Henry Miller, MD, in 1849; he became AMA president in 1859. Samuel D. Gross, the president in 1868, had published in 1839 the first American textbook on pathological anatomy.

The founding of *JAMA*

In keeping with the overall emphasis on scientific issues, probably no action taken during the AMA's first 50 years of existence would equal in its long-term importance the decision to found the *Journal of the American Medical Association* in 1880. Until that time, the Association had published the transactions of the annual meeting each year. The leading proponent of change that year was the AMA's president, Lewis A. Sayre, MD, an outspoken admirer of the *British Medical Journal* published by the British Medical Association. He envisioned a new AMA weekly publication as a tool for acquiring new members, as a means of disseminating educational information, and as a source of revenue.

By 1882, it had become time to act. A five-member committee on publications estimated the annual cost of printing a weekly journal would be some $15,000 a year. With approximately 90,000 physicians in the United States, it was estimated that if a mere 3000 new members were attracted, the costs of publication would be met.

At the same time, the Association was in the process of forming a Board of Trustees to manage the day-to-day affairs of the organization. Perhaps not surprisingly, Dr Nathan Davis was chosen as the first chairman. However, he stepped down in 1883 to become *JAMA*'s first editor, and Volume 1, No. 1, with 32 pages, appeared on July 14, 1883.

Dr Davis would go on to serve as editor until 1888, when he was succeeded by John S. Hamilton, MD, formerly the supervising surgeon general of the Marine Hospital Service. One of Dr Hamilton's early editorials noted: "There are a little more than 80,000 persons practicing medicine in the United States, of whom more than 60,000 are regular practitioners. When one-third of the regular profession are members of the American Medical Association, we can have the strongest organization and the best medical journal in the world." Dr Hamilton, John H. Hollister, MD, and J. C. Culbertson, MD, edited the publication until 1899, when George H. Simmons, MD, began a 25-year tenure that was marked by some of the publication's greatest advances.

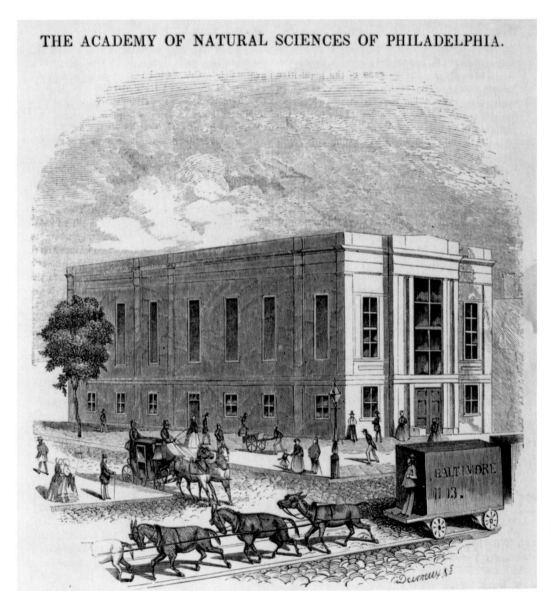

THE ACADEMY OF NATURAL SCIENCES OF PHILADELPHIA.

Early view of the Philadelphia Academy of Natural Sciences, where the AMA was founded.

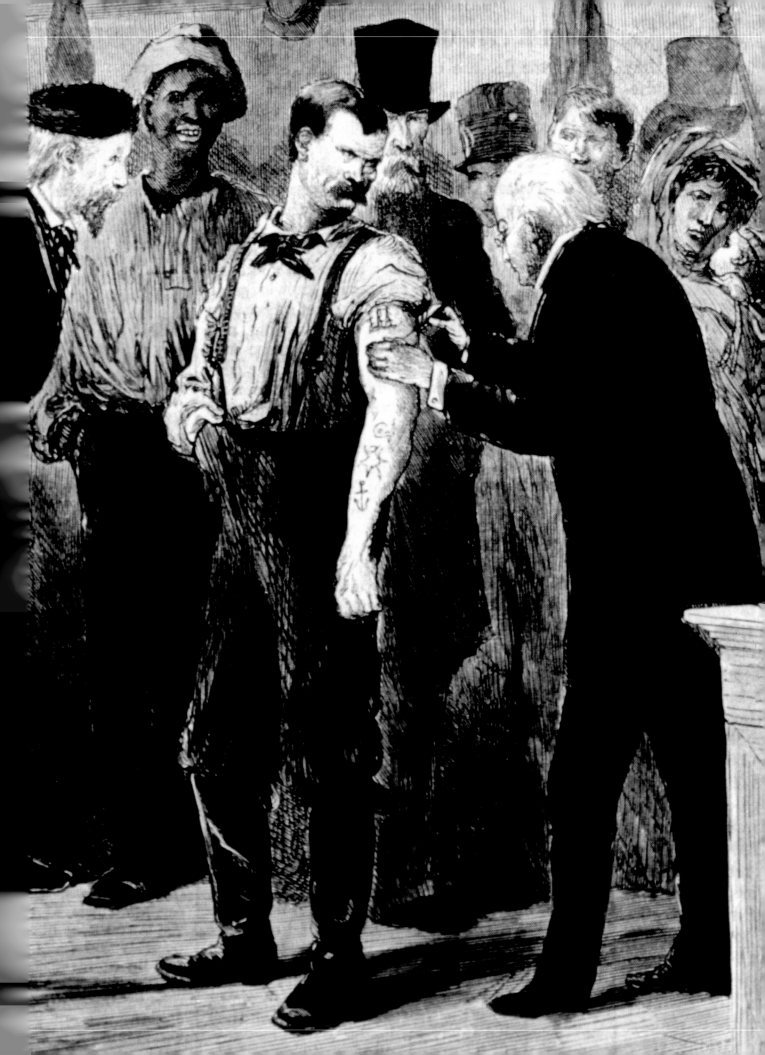

The first 50 years

Meanwhile, there was the AMA's 50th birthday to observe. The semicentennial meeting, held in Philadelphia in 1897, was attended by President William McKinley. The AMA president, Nicholas Senn, MD, a world-renowned surgeon from Chicago, gave the participants this "glimpse of the future":

> *"Fifty years of steady growth has made the American Medical Association strong. It has passed the experimental stage; it has done a great deal in advancing and diffusing medical knowledge and in the prevention, alleviation, and cure of disease. It is the recognized final tribunal which directs and controls all other medical societies and medical educational institutions. It is the final Court of Appeals to which the regular practitioners and the public can look with confidence for the enforcement of a pure discipline and needed protection. It is the highest postgraduate medical institution in this country which without tuition provides a course of instruction annually of a scientific and practical character, well adapted for the busy practitioner, from which every one returns with a firm determination to do more and better work."*

He added these prophetic words:

> *"It is difficult to foretell the possibilities of the second half of the first century of the existence of the Association. It is, however, safe to predict that when the first centennial celebration will be held in this city fifty years from now the membership will have increased from 9,000 to 75,000 or 100,000 and our official organ at that time will be recognized the world over as the most enterprising and best medical journal."*

As the end of the century neared and the AMA began its second 50 years, there was, in fact, much justified cause for optimism.

The growth of AMA membership, the financial stability provided by the growth of *JAMA,* and increased public and professional respect for the Association had placed it in its strongest position ever. A "critical mass" had been achieved. As the century ended, the AMA was poised to embark on an ambitious course. One major effort would be to solidify its position as the ethical standard-bearer for the entire profession.

Facing page: Smallpox vaccination at a clinic for the poor, 1873.

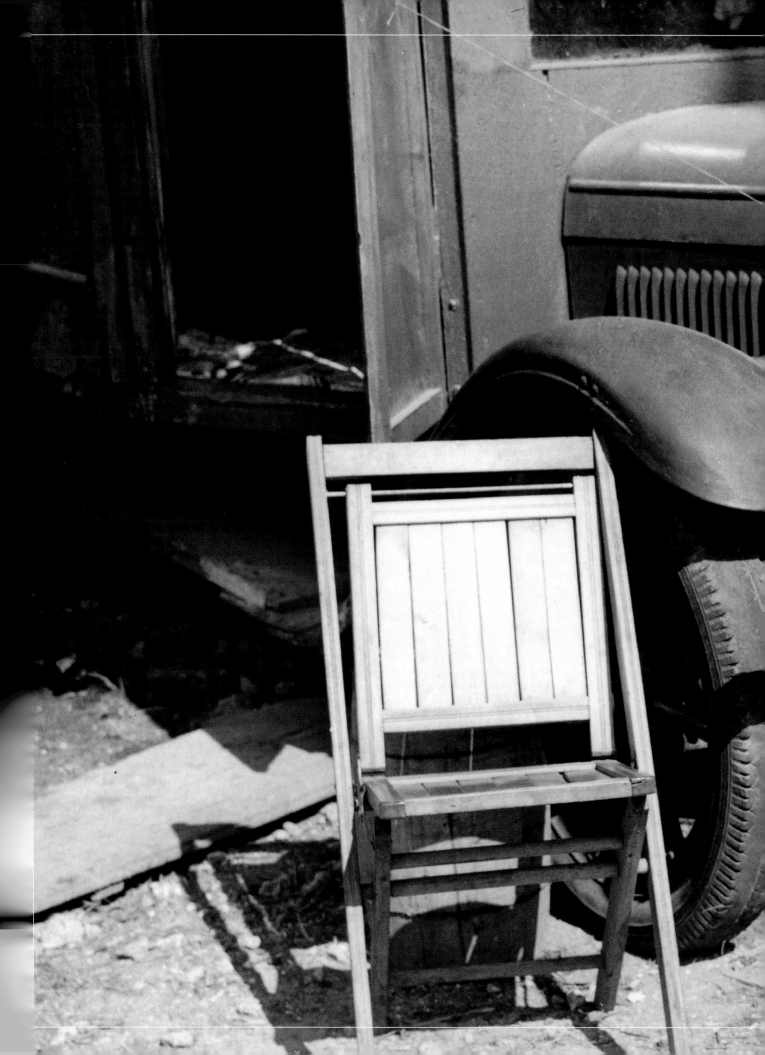

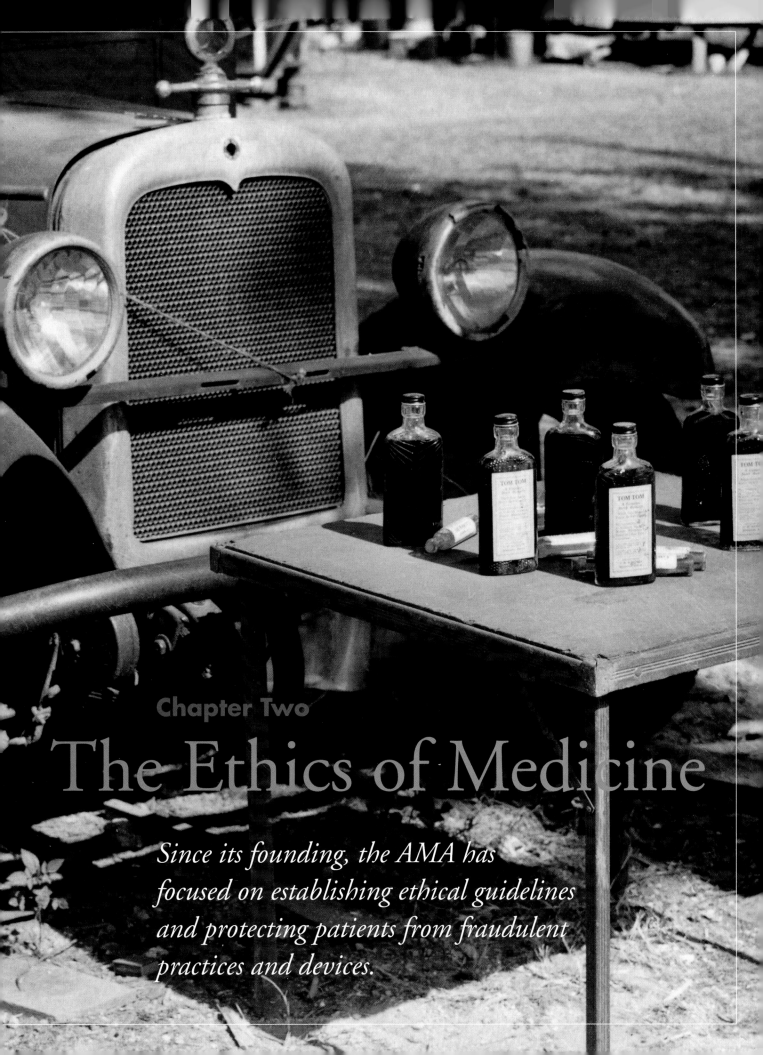

Chapter Two

The Ethics of Medicine

*Since its founding, the AMA has
focused on establishing ethical guidelines
and protecting patients from fraudulent
practices and devices.*

2

The Ethics of Medicine

From the very beginning of the American Medical Association, the profession's ethics were a primary concern. While time, medical advances, government regulation, and cultural changes have changed the issues — and made them more complicated — this tradition of high ethical standards remains one of medicine's proudest heritages.

When the American Medical Association was founded in 1847, a committee was named to prepare a code of medical ethics for the profession. After considerable study, the committee recommended the Code of Medical Ethics prepared in 1803 by Thomas Percival. Dr Percival had written his code for the guidance of the surgeons and physicians at England's Manchester University, at which he had an appointment. His Code compiled the approved customs, rules, and practices prevalent in England at the time.

The AMA committee reported that, on examining a great number of codes of ethics adopted by different professional societies in the United States, it was found that they were all based on that by Dr Percival, and that the phrases of this writer were preserved, to a considerable extent, in all of them. "Believing that language which had been so often examined and adopted must possess the greatest of merits for such a document as the present, clearness and precision, and having no ambition for the honours of authorship, the Committee which prepared this code have followed a similar course and

Overleaf: Before the AMA helped stop sales of patent medicines, vendors often sold their wares directly from a car or truck to the public. This card-table with patent medicine bottles was photographed in 1939.

have carefully preserved the words of Percival wherever they convey the precepts it is wished to inculcate. A few of the sections are in the words of the late Dr [Benjamin] Rush, and one or two sentences are from other writers."

This 1847 Code remained basically intact for more than a century, although there were some minor changes in 1903 and the title was changed to the Principles of Medical Ethics.

For the first decade of the AMA's existence, the Code of Medical Ethics was an informational document, advising individual physicians of acceptable standards of conduct. Initially, there was no mechanism for enforcement, but in 1858, the first Committee on Ethics was established. This committee was appointed by the AMA president at each meeting and sat only for the duration of the meeting.

One of the first issues addressed by the Committee was the role of women in medical practice, and in 1868, the Committee sanctioned the role of regularly educated and otherwise well-qualified female physicians.

The question of homeopathic and eclectic practitioners came up in 1870, and the Committee stated that such "cult practice" was "plainly in violation" of the Code. The issue of cult practice led to a long and divisive battle in New York. In 1882, the New York Medical Society adopted its own simplified code and was then expelled from the AMA; the New York State Society subsequently achieved representation, and the conflict was not resolved until 1903, when the revised Principles left the issue of homeopathy to local societies for decision.

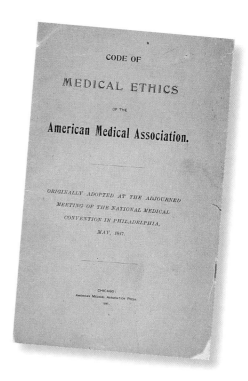

An 1897 reproduction of the AMA's original Code of Medical Ethics, published in 1847.

Evolving over 150 years,
AMA's ethical standards
have guided the profession.

In 1873, Dr Nathan S. Davis — 26 years after he helped found the AMA — proposed formation of the Association's Judicial Council to succeed the Committee on Ethics. The 21-member committee would take cognizance of and decide "all questions of an ethical or judicial character that might arise in connection with the Association."

The 1901 reorganization of the AMA established the Judicial Council as the AMA's judicial body. However, the 21-member body was proving unwieldy, and in 1911 the Bylaws were amended to reduce the size of the Council to five members, one to be nominated by the president each year and confirmed by the House of Delegates. (This selection process continues today, although the size of the Council has been increased to nine members.)

The first chair of the five-member Council was Frank Billings, MD, a prominent Chicagoan, and the new Council immediately drafted a revised Principles of Medical Ethics, which was adopted by the House of Delegates in 1912. The Council also acted immediately to condemn the secret division of fees among physicians and the payment of commissions, and called for amendments to the Constitution and Bylaws opposing the patenting of drugs and medical instruments.

The Judicial Council addressed economics as well as ethics

Two years later, the Judicial Council submitted a report that opposed advertising by physicians as quackery. It was not until the 1920s, however, that the Council became heavily involved in the economics of medical practice. In 1922, the Council took aim at group medical practice clinics that obtained patients by advertising and developed an amendment to

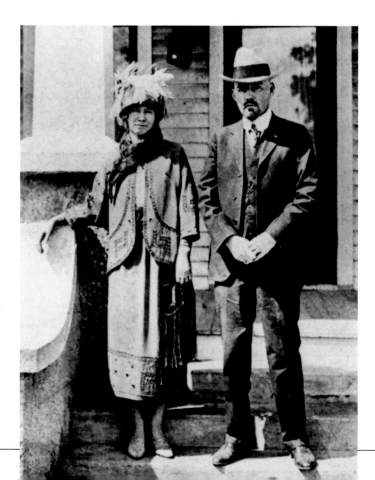

John Brinkley (with his wife in the 1920s) was a long-time AMA target. He used radio advertising to tout his "goat gland" surgery for impotence.

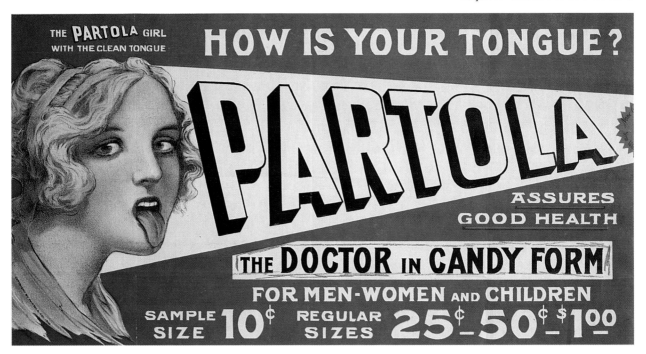

THE **PARTOLA** GIRL
WITH THE CLEAN TONGUE

HOW IS YOUR TONGUE?

PARTOLA

ASSURES
GOOD HEALTH

THE **DOCTOR** IN **CANDY FORM**

FOR MEN-WOMEN AND CHILDREN

SAMPLE SIZE **10**¢ REGULAR SIZES **25**¢–**50**¢–**$1**⁰⁰

**Home remedies
promised relief
from ailments
ranging from
trivial to serious.**

the Principles outlawing the solicitation of patients by physicians — a policy
that remained in effect until the new Principles were adopted in 1980. In
1930 came a directive on corporate medical practice, which stated:

> "…such practice is detrimental to the best interests of scientific medicine and
> of the people themselves. When medical service is made impersonal, when the
> humanities of medicine are removed, when the coldness and automaticity of the
> machine are substituted for the humane interest inherent in individual service
> and the professional and scientific independence of the individual physician,
> the greatest incentive to scientific improvement will be destroyed and the
> public will be poorly served."

A 1934 Council statement — in the height of the Depression — endorsed
the philosophy of providing services for all needy patients and refusal to
accept payment from the government, warning that the "adoption of a
principle of service only when paid for would be the greatest step toward
socialized medicine and shortly state medicine…."

However, the reality of the Depression was that many physicians in fact
could not afford to provide charity services if there was the possibility
of reimbursement by a third party. Therefore, a 1934 amendment to
the Principles made it unethical for a physician to dispose of his or her
services to any lay body, organization, group, or individual under conditions
that would permit any of these third parties to receive a profit on the
doctor's services.

The end of the Depression and the war years slowed the activities of the Council — as well as virtually all of organized medicine not devoted to the war effort — and it was not until the 1950s that major ethical conflicts resurfaced.

The Principles guided new resolutions in the 1950s

In 1952, the House of Delegates adopted a Council report condemning as fee splitting "the suggestion made by some hospitals that physicians who utilize hospital facilities should pay to the hospital a percentage of the fees they receive from patients while being cared for in the hospital." The next year, the Council addressed the salaried employment of physicians — particularly anesthesiologists, radiologists, and physiatrists — stating that "the acceptance of a salary by a physician does not of itself constitute unethical conduct."

A 1954 statement targeted ophthalmology, stating that "it is unethical for ophthalmologists to profit from the sale of glasses. Ophthalmologists cannot derive income from merchandising and still be considered on a professional level." A year later, a resolution from the Section on Ophthalmology was adopted that made it unethical for a physician to teach in a school of optometry or to lecture to optometrists. (This statement would be rescinded a decade later after the filing of an antitrust suit against the AMA.)

The 1920s "Spectro-Chrome" claimed to cure almost any disease by exposing the patient to pure, intense colored light.

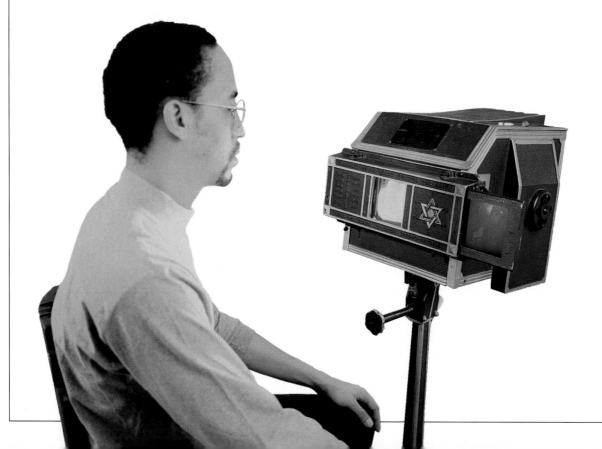

Facing page: This ad for Milton makes a variety of claims for the product but fails to mention a single ingredient.

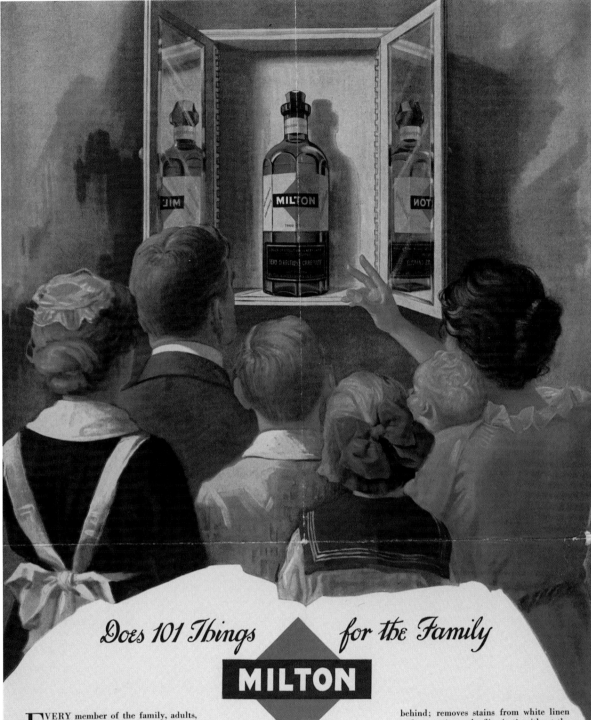

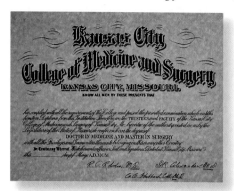

Typical "diploma mill" degree. This school opened in 1916 and was closed by the authorities in 1926.

A major revision of the Principles took place in 1957, after 2 years of debate by the House of Delegates. The old Principles of about 4000 words were replaced by a 500-word document with only 10 brief sections. The goal was to eliminate specific regulations governing particular conduct, leaving only fundamental ethical principles from which it could be reasoned whether a particular act was unethical. This change gave the Judicial Council broad rule-making authority. The Council could issue ethical pronouncements on complex issues — on human experimentation, termination of life support, etc — without the necessity of securing House of Delegates approval for an amendment to the Principles.

The AMA responds to the changing health care system

By the 1970s, the federal government's involvement in the health care industry had become a major issue for all of medicine, including the AMA and its ethical activities. The AMA's Principles provided that the physician "should not solicit patients" and "not dispose of his services under terms or conditions which tend to interfere with or impair the free and complete exercise of his medical judgment." This was interpreted as a ban on advertising and disapproval of "contract" practice, and on December 19, 1975, the Federal Trade Commission (FTC) charged the AMA with illegally restricting its members from advertising and soliciting patients and interfering with the relationship between physicians and such entities as health maintenance organizations and prepaid plans.

An FTC administrative law judge found the AMA's policy anticompetitive and an unreasonable restraint of trade. The full FTC issued an order requiring the AMA to stop such restraints — except with respect to "false and deceptive" advertising. The AMA appealed, and the case wound up taking several years to make its way through the federal court system. A federal appeals court upheld the FTC order after clarifying it to protect such activities as peer review of the fee practices of physicians who engage in a pattern of excessive fees. The order was affirmed by the Supreme Court in 1982 — by a 4-4 tie vote.

Legal and ethical controversies lead to **a new code of ethics** *within the American Medical Association.*

As the antitrust litigation was wending its way through the courts, the AMA also was taking action. In 1978, a young New Jersey surgeon, James S. Todd, MD, was named to chair an ad hoc committee that would draft a proposed new Code of Ethics. Dr Todd had been a member of the House for only 2 years, although he was well known through participation in the AMA's speakers bureau. Committee members including Jean Crum, MD, of California; Henrietta Herbolsheimer, MD, of Illinois; and Carroll Witten, MD, of Kentucky, joined him in 2 years of effort in which they talked with ethicists, held hearings involving practicing physicians, and prepared countless drafts of the proposed code. By the time of the 1980 Annual Meeting of the House of Delegates, the report was ready for final consideration.

More than revision — drafting a new Code of Ethics

When the House of Delegates convened in July, the fate of the Todd committee's product was very much in doubt. Some AMA officials and senior staff believed that amending the existing Principles was a better way to go, and the committee had resisted pressures to withdraw or delay its

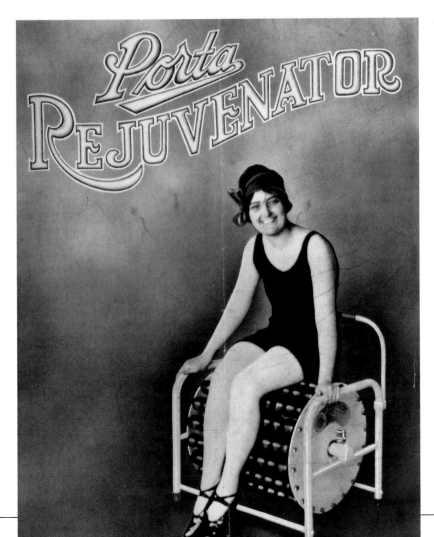

"Rejuvenation" was a popular theme in health fraud ads. The AMA has battled tirelessly against the marketing of fraudulent devices.

report. At the reference committee hearing and on the floor of the House itself, Dr Todd put forth the rationale for change in forceful, eloquent terms. "Revisions of ethics have occurred on at least four previous occasions," he said, "and each time the stimulus was either changes within the profession or within history. Looking at history then, there is no question that medical ethics can, should and do change and with the heightening pressure upon the Association, there is fairly general agreement that some change once again is necessary. The issue remaining is how much."

Limited change — modifying the existing code to bring it into compliance with the FTC's demands — was not a viable option to Dr Todd, because the result would be a patchwork document that would require constant revision. He then got to the crux of his argument:

"No one should expect any Principles of Medical Ethics to remain unchanged forever, but by responding in a consistent fashion to a rapidly expanding and changing profession and society, physicians can demonstrate their dedication to their patients…These Principles accurately reflect a proper contemporary ethical stance for the profession; they are acceptable to a significant portion of the profession; they are supported by the Judicial Council; they conform to present legal requirements; they are a firm foundation upon which further interpretation and expansions can be built; they can withstand further changes within the profession and society and they are strong and patient oriented."

The time had come, he said, to "face up to the real issues. Do we simply reach a defiant accommodation or do we seize the opportunity to demonstrate our deep commitment to our patients by producing Ethics reflecting a professional and social reality? A profession so quick to accept scientific change should not be reluctant to accept the professional and social consequences of that change."

Although political insiders the evening before had pronounced the ad hoc committee report doomed, Dr Todd's eloquence carried the day. The report carried, receiving 195 votes — 12 more than the required two-thirds majority.

At the same time, Dr Todd, backed by his state medical society, had decided to seek election to the AMA Board of Trustees at that same meeting of the delegates ("I figured it was win/win or lose/lose," he would recall later), and the adoption of the new Code would assure his election. He would move up to vice chair of the Board by 1986 when the AMA's executive vice president, James H. Sammons, MD, tapped him to be the deputy executive vice president.

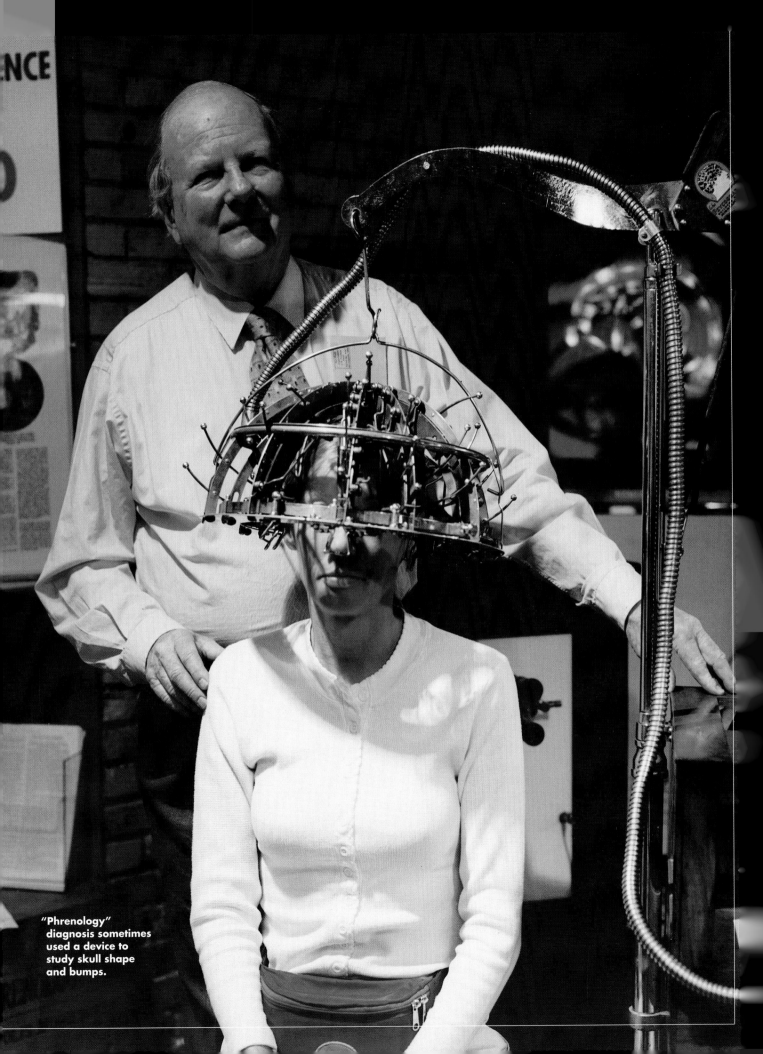

"Phrenology"
diagnosis sometimes
used a device to
study skull shape
and bumps.

Principles of Medical Ethics

Following is the text of the Principles of Medical Ethics, drafted by the special committee chaired by James S. Todd, MD, and adopted by the House of Delegates in July 1980.

Preamble:

The medical profession has long subscribed to a body of ethical statements developed primarily for the benefit of the patient. As a member of this profession, a physician must recognize responsibility not only to the patient, but also to society, to other health professionals, and to self. The following principles adopted by the American Medical Association are not laws, but standards of conduct which define the essentials of honorable behavior for the physician.

I. **A physician shall be dedicated to providing competent medical service with compassion and respect for human dignity.**

II. **A physician shall deal honestly with patients and colleagues, and strive to expose those physicians deficient in character or competence, or who engage in fraud or deception.**

III. **A physician shall respect the law and also recognize a responsibility to seek changes in those requirements which are contrary to the best interests of the patient.**

IV. **A physician shall respect the rights of patients, of colleagues, and of other health professionals, and shall safeguard patient confidences within the constraints of the law.**

V. **A physician shall continue to study, apply and advance scientific knowledge, make relevant information available to patients, colleagues, and the public, obtain consultation, and use the talents of other health professionals when indicated.**

VI. **A physician shall, in the provision of appropriate patient care, except in emergencies, be free to choose whom to serve, with whom to associate, and the environment in which to provide medical services.**

VII. **A physician shall recognize a responsibility to participate in activities contributing to an improved community.**

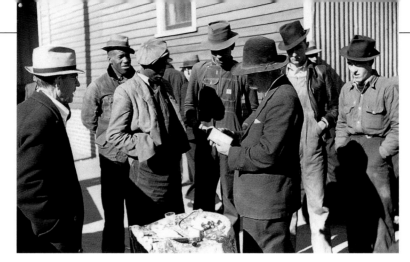

A patent medicine ("snake oil") salesman in 1939.

The AMA's 1980 Code has proven to be a sound framework as the Council on Ethical and Judicial Affairs (the new name for the Judicial Council as of 1985) wrests with the complex issues that now are a part of the practice of medicine. The Council's "Current Opinions" fill some 50 pages in the *AMA Policy Compendium,* broadly grouped into such areas as social policy issues, interprofessional relations, hospital relations, confidentiality, advertising, communications media relations, fees and charges, and gifts from industry.

Still fresh — The Principles and "Current Opinions"

Some of the issues the Council now is addressing — end of life decisions, genetic medicine, the challenges of managed care, professionalism — involve difficult moral, ethical, and legal judgments. The Council and the AMA, relying on the Principles and the wealth of material in the "Current Opinions," have become recognized not only by the medical profession but by the public, the media, and the courts as the principal arbiters as society wrestles with the complex issues of the 1990s.

In fact, while ethical issues were one of the foundations for the AMA's beginnings, they have become even more important today. The AMA has recognized this and is placing greater emphasis on its ethical activities than ever before. A prominent Harvard ethicist joined the Association's staff in 1996, and the AMA's sesquicentennial observance in 1997 was scheduled to include a major national conference on ethics in Philadelphia, the city of the AMA's founding.

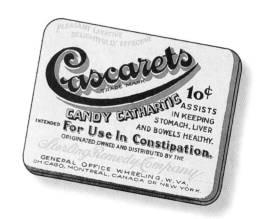

Even "candy" was reputed to have therapeutic properties.

The visionary founders of the American Medical Association in 1847 were precisely on target in their emphasis on ethical issues for their new organization. Yet it would have been impossible for them to imagine the changes in medicine, in science and technology, and in society that would occur in the next 150 years. Nevertheless, they put in place the framework for an ethical system that has allowed the AMA today to become the acknowledged leader in this field.

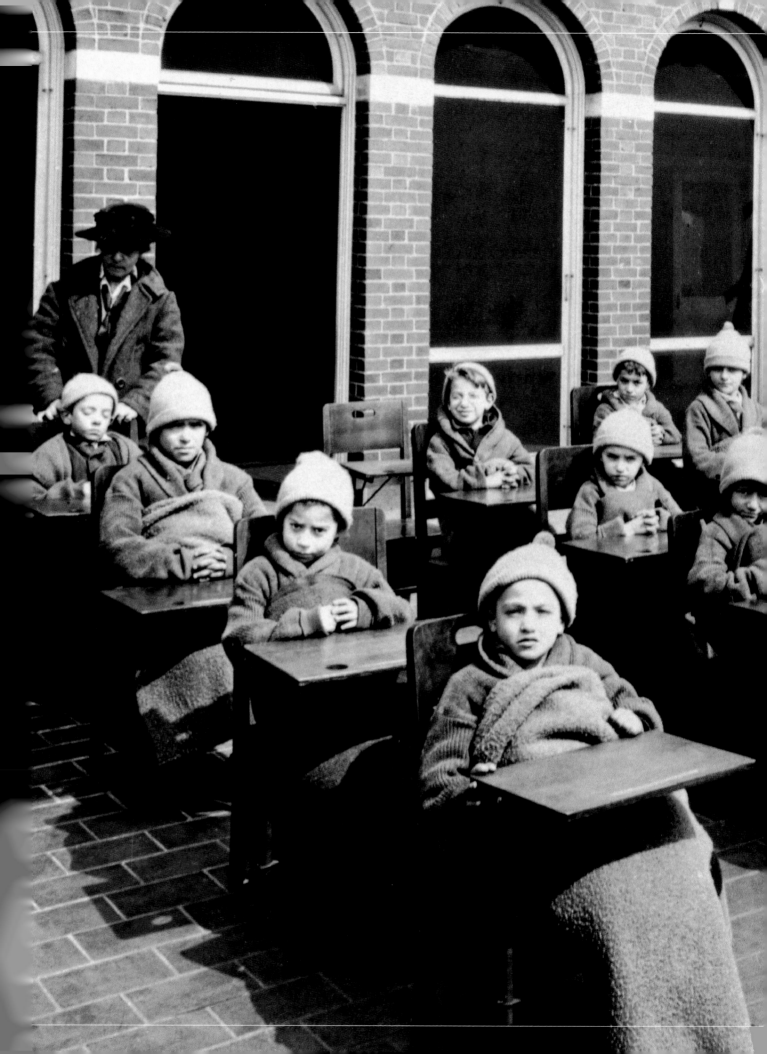

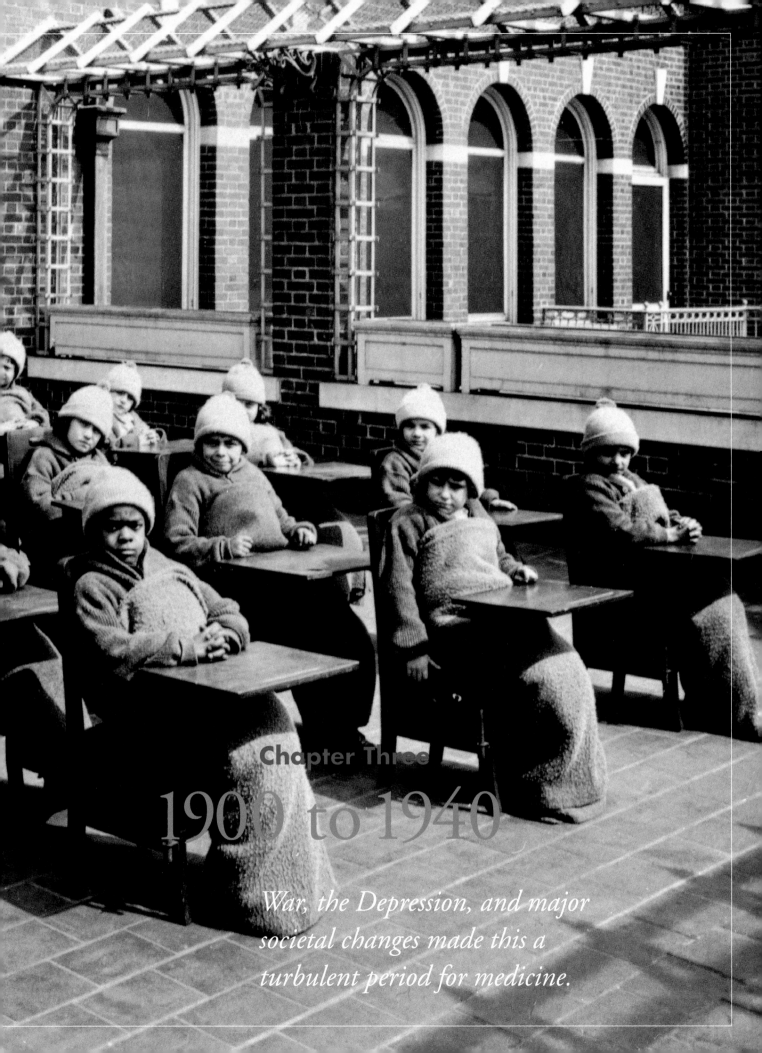

Chapter Three
1900 to 1940

War, the Depression, and major societal changes made this a turbulent period for medicine.

3

1900 to 1940

The turn of the century coincided with a period of rapid transition for the American Medical Association, which in a few short years was to transform itself into a powerful voice on all health topics — a voice that would be listened to by the profession, by the public, and by policymakers.

Two major steps actually occurred in 1899. One was the appointment of George H. Simmons, MD, as the editor of the *Journal of the American Medical Association.* Dr Simmons would serve in that capacity for 25 years, during which he would transform *JAMA* into one of the world's most respected medical journals. The publication's success had a salutary effect on many other AMA activities; the revenue generated by advertising and subscriptions would fund other Association programs without the need for raising dues, which were $10. Also in 1899, the AMA created a Committee on National Legislation, marking the organization's first step toward establishment of a national presence in health care policy.

At the turn of the century AMA membership stood at approximately 9000, among some 100,000 "regular physicians" in the United States; the circulation of *JAMA* had reached 15,000. The AMA held its annual meeting that year in Atlantic City and appointed a Committee on Organization to examine the AMA's structure and as well as the structure of the constituent organizations. That committee was made up of one member from each state and territory represented in the AMA; it appointed a three-member Committee on Reorganization to turn recommendations into specific policy.

The Committee on Reorganization — J. N. McCormack, MD, of Bowling Green, Ky; P. Maxwell Foshay, MD, of Cleveland; and *JAMA*'s Dr Simmons — produced in 1901 a set of constitutional amendments that transformed the AMA into an organization very similar to the one that exists today. Under the 1901 constitutional revisions, AMA membership would be granted to all members of local medical societies affiliated with state medical societies who applied for membership, supplied certification of good standing, and paid the annual fee. The Association's governing body would be a new House of Delegates made up of representatives of state medical societies (plus representatives from the military and from AMA sections). States' representation in the House of Delegates would be based on one delegate per 500 state medical society members, with total membership in the House capped at 150.

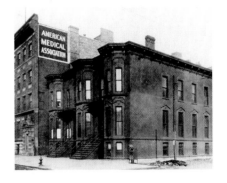

(A note from *The History of the American Medical Association 1847 to 1947*, by Morris Fishbein, MD: "The Committee on Reorganization had been voted $400 for its expenses, but the total bills represented $416.89. This gave great concern to the Board of Trustees, which eventually decided to give $400 to the chairman and let him argue it out with the other two members.")

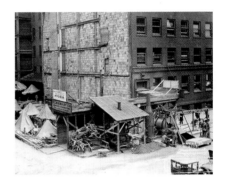

Meanwhile, other major changes were taking place. In 1902, the AMA purchased three lots in Chicago, at the corner of Grand and Dearborn — the site that would serve as the AMA's home at 535 N Dearborn for nearly 90 years. The Council on Medical Education was founded in 1904 and immediately set out to raise the level of training for physicians. In 1905 came the formation of the Council on Pharmacy, which would establish standards for drug manufacturing and advertising, as well as conduct a widely publicized war on quack remedies, dubious patent medicines, and other nostrums. A year later, the AMA established its own chemical laboratory to analyze medicines and drugs.

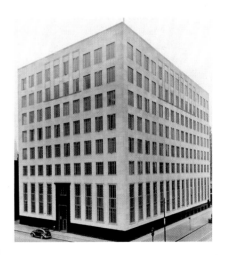

The evolution of AMA's headquarters (from top to bottom): the original building at 535 N Dearborn (ca 1905); 1922 construction of the "new" building; and 535 N Dearborn as it looked in the 1940s.

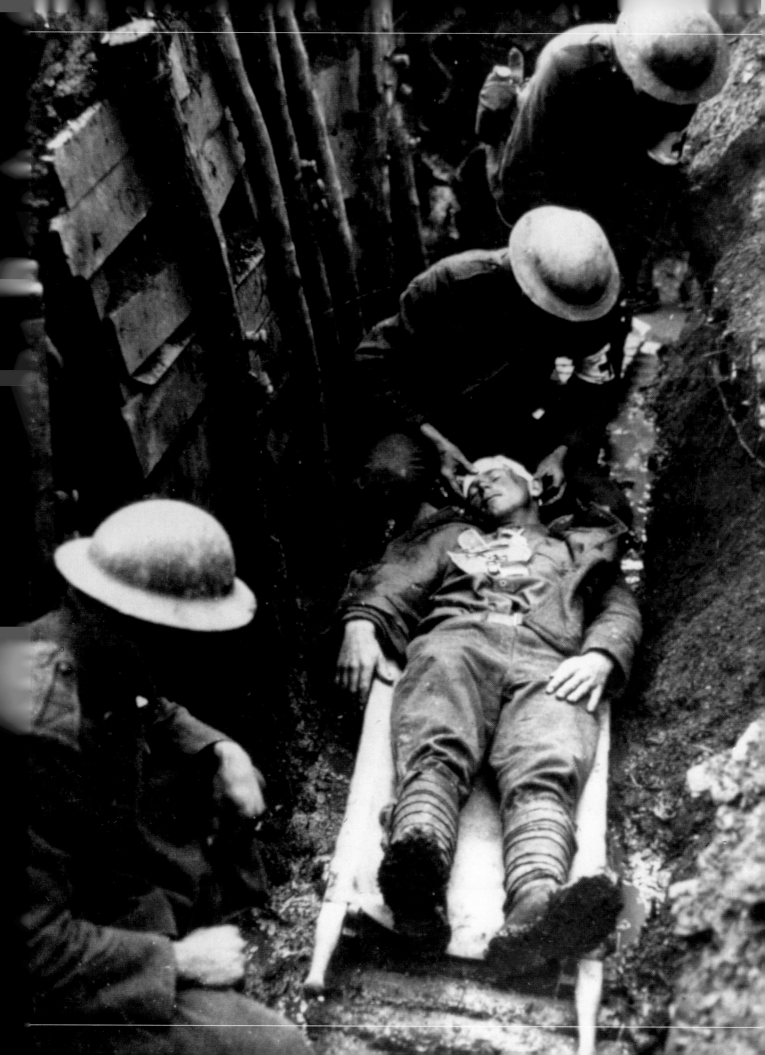

The war on quackery took another step forward in 1913 when the AMA established a "propaganda department" — it would probably be named something else today — to make the media and the public aware of health fraud and quackery problems. That year also saw an event that would affect the course of the organization for the next 50 years, although no one knew it at the time: Morris Fishbein, MD, fresh out of Chicago's Rush Medical School, joined the staff of *JAMA*. Also in 1913, the AMA first expressed an interest in what was then known as "sickness insurance," which at that time was available in some European countries.

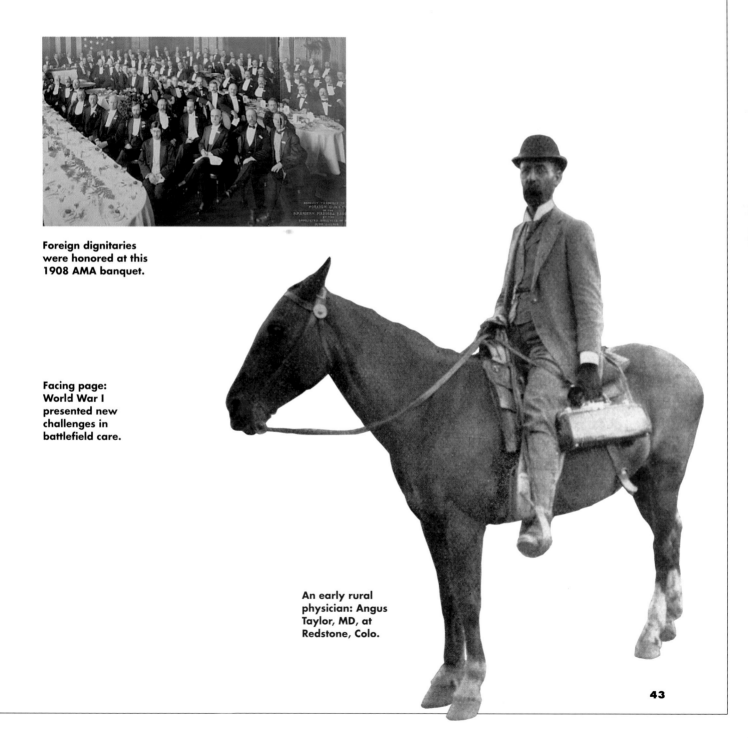

Foreign dignitaries were honored at this 1908 AMA banquet.

Facing page: World War I presented new challenges in battlefield care.

An early rural physician: Angus Taylor, MD, at Redstone, Colo.

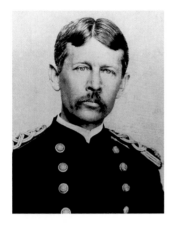

Walter Reed, MD, whose pioneering work demonstrated transmission of malaria by mosquitoes.

However, sickness insurance was to occupy much of the AMA's time and energy for several years. In 1917, the House of Delegates approved a resolution authorizing the Council on Health and Public Instruction "in the interests of both the wage earners and the medical profession" to "continue to study and to make reports on the future development of social insurance legislation and to cooperate, when possible, in the molding of these laws that the health of the community may be properly safeguarded and the interests of the medical profession protected." Such legislation, the resolution stated, should "provide for freedom of choice of physician by the insured; payment of the physician in proportion to the amount of work done; the separation of the functions of medical office supervision from the function of daily care of the sick; and adequate representation of the medical profession on the appropriate administrative bodies."

War concerns supercede social insurance

This policy statement was to be repudiated in a few years, but first the AMA — along with the rest of the United States — turned its attention to the war in Europe. The AMA complied with a War Department request and organized the establishment of medical boards in every state to examine the health of men called up for the military draft. On April 7, 1917, *JAMA* noted that war was imminent and called on members of the medical profession to step forward as volunteers. William J. Mayo, MD, had become chairman of the American Physicians for Medical Preparedness,

The World War I American Ambulance Hospital in Paris; the ambulances were donated by Henry Ford.

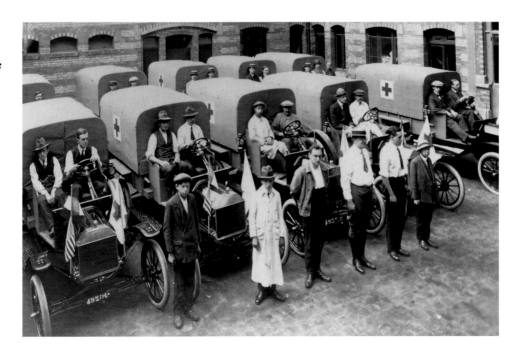

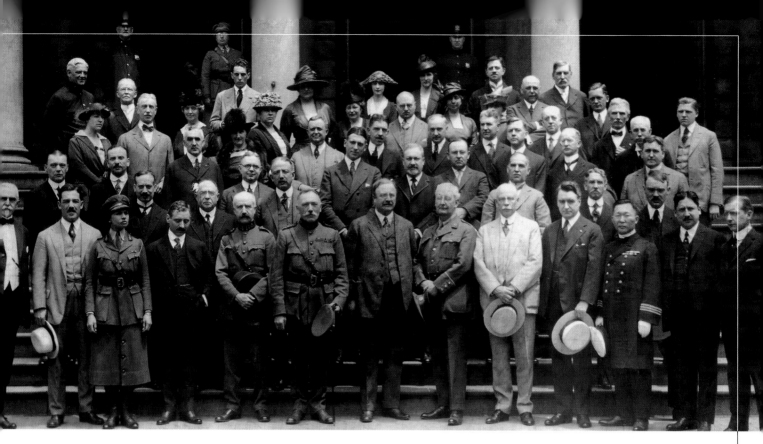

which had organized nine-member committees in each state and many county committees. While this organization had no formal tie to the AMA, it relied on *JAMA* and the AMA's biographic files for much of its function.

The April 21, 1917, issue of *JAMA* (the United States had just formally entered the war) included a form for application to the Army Medical Corps and for appointment in the reserve officers corps. Throughout the war, *JAMA* would continue to support the war effort, appealing for volunteers, publishing each week the orders to medical officers, and in general carrying out exhaustive coverage of military medical affairs. The June 1, 1918, *JAMA* carried a complete list of the civilian physicians in the military service, tabulated by counties and states.

William Gorgas, MD, controlled yellow fever to make possible construction of the Panama Canal.

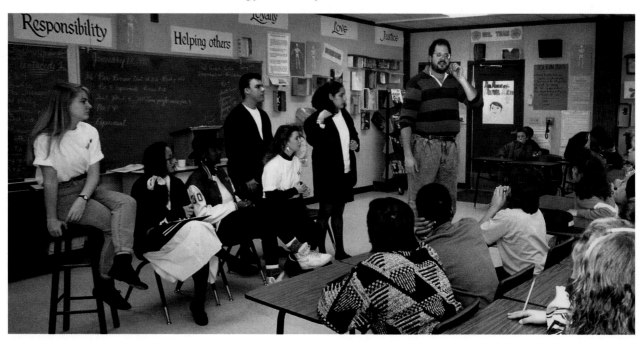

From its modest beginnings, the Auxiliary (later Alliance) expanded to offer school programs like this one in Fresno, Calif.

The relatively short duration of US involvement in the war had minimized its impact on the home front and on medical education. Nevertheless, 35,000 physicians took part, among them many of the AMA's leaders. Dr Fishbein's *History* notes that in 1918, all five members of the Council on Health and Public Instruction and its secretary were in military service. Consequently, the council's 1918 report was brief and "the entire section on social insurance had disappeared. It is interesting to think what might have happened relating to social insurance if the war had not intervened."

Within a couple of years, however, the issue had resurfaced. Several state medical journals had assailed the Council's earlier position, and at the 1920 meeting, the House of Delegates adopted the following resolution:

"The American Medical Association declares its opposition to the institution of any plan embodying the system of compulsory contributory insurance against illness, or any other plan of compulsory insurance which provides for medical service to be rendered contributors or their dependents, provided, controlled or regulated by any state or the federal government."

This policy remained on the AMA's books for decades; it did not, however, still the debate over the government's proper role in health care.

The House of Delegates in 1922 declared the AMA's "opposition to all forms of 'state medicine' because of the ultimate harm that would come to the public weal through such form of medical practice." (At the same meeting, a proposal that group insurance be provided for all AMA employees was sent to the Board of Trustees. However, it was some 20 years before such coverage was provided.)

New developments in the 1920s and 1930s

Two other events took place in 1922 that would have long-term effects on medicine. The House of Delegates approved a resolution from Texas that established the Woman's Auxiliary to the American Medical Association. Its mission would be to "extend the aims of the medical profession through the wives of doctors to the various women's organizations, which look to the advancement in health and education; also to assist in entertainment at all medical conventions and to promote acquaintanceship among doctors' families that closer professional fellowship may exist." More than 70 years later, the Auxiliary — now the AMA Alliance — has 55,000 members, a long, distinguished record of civic and public health accomplishments, and a number of male members.

Also at the 1922 meeting, the House of Delegates urged the Board to proceed as rapidly as possible with the development of a journal for the public. This would become *Hygeia* (later *Today's Health*), for many years a highly successful health education mechanism with widespread consumer acceptance. In 1924, the AMA also began radio broadcasts of health information for the public.

The 1920s also saw significant changes in AMA's staff leadership. Dr Simmons retired as editor and general manager. His duties were divided between Olin West, MD, general manager, and Dr Fishbein, who began his long career as *JAMA* editor.

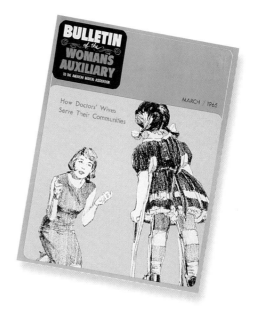

This 1965 issue of the *Bulletin of the Woman's Auxiliary* — as did many others — featured community service activities of physicians' spouses.

Public health education **is a proud tradition for** *the AMA and its Alliance.*

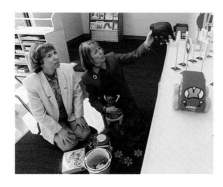

An Idaho Alliance project in the 1990s for mothers who are inmates in a women's prison.

In 1927 came the appointment of a national Committee on the Costs of Medical Care that would have far-reaching effects. The Committee was independent of the AMA and was sponsored by a foundation. However, its chairman was Ray Lyman Wilbur, MD, AMA president in 1923 and chairman of the Council on Medical Education and Hospitals, on which he served from 1929 to 1945. He was also president of Stanford University and President Hoover's Secretary of the Interior.

The Committee on the Costs of Medical Care published its final report in late 1932, and the AMA's response was quick and forceful. Noting that the Committee's majority report supported the growth of contract practice while the minority report opposed it, Dr Fishbein (with the Board's blessing) wrote in *JAMA*:

" These two reports represent...the difference between incitement to revolution and a desire for gradual evolution based on analysis and study. The majority report urges reorganization of medical practice, the development of centers, insurance; if necessary taxation to provide funds; expansion of public health services. The minority is willing to test any plan that may be offered if it conforms to the medical conception of what is known to be good medical practice. Indeed, the minority recommends 'that methods be given careful trial which can rightly be fitted into our present institutions and agencies without interfering with the fundamentals of medical practice.' One seems to hear that famous medical aphorism that has come down through the centuries: 'Prove all things; hold fast to that which is good.'"

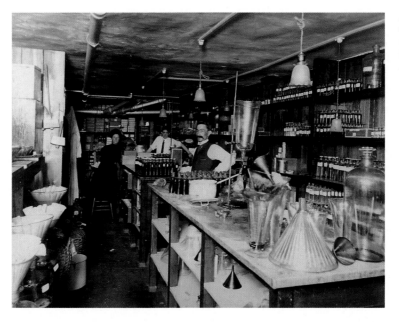

Many drugs were formulated in local pharmacies like this one, around 1910.

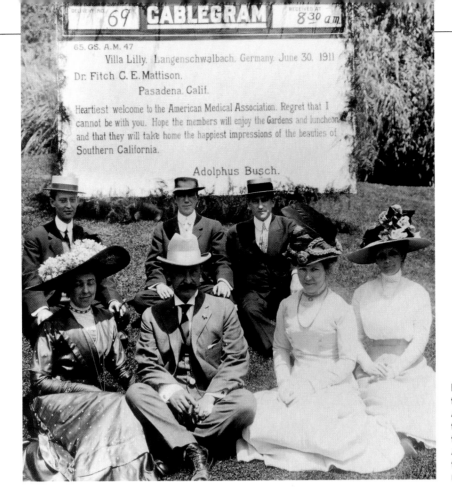

CABLEGRAM

69   8 30 a.m.

65. GS. A.M. 47
        Villa Lilly, Langenschwalbach, Germany, June 30, 1911
Dr. Fitch C. E. Mattison,
        Pasadena, Calif.

Heartiest welcome to the American Medical Association. Regret that I
cannot be with you. Hope the members will enjoy the Gardens and luncheon,
and that they will take home the happiest impressions of the beauties of
Southern California.

        Adolphus Busch.

Improved rail travel broadened AMA's vistas; these attendees traveled to Los Angeles for the 1911 AMA meeting.

Social changes bring medical issues

The rise of Hitler's totalitarian regime in Europe in the early 1930s created another problem for medicine in this country, as a steady stream of refugee physicians arrived in the United States. This led the Council on Medical Education and Hospitals to draw up a list of foreign medical schools whose training might produce acceptable physicians, for the guidance of state licensing boards. The supply of physicians in this country was still feeling the effects of the activities of the Flexner Report and the AMA's attacks on diploma mills; there were only 75 medical schools in existence in 1930, down from 162 in 1904. However, by 1931, AMA membership had passed 100,000 for the first time.

Also, the Volstead Act — Prohibition — was a long-running contentious issue for medicine and the AMA. Alcohol was available by prescription, and many physicians were pressured by patients to write such prescriptions. During 1931, the permits of 977 physicians were revoked for illegal prescribing; one physician estimated that 90% of the prescriptions written for alcohol were used for beverage and not for scientific treatment of disease. *JAMA* waged an ongoing war against this type of prescribing, going so far as to point out, in Dr Fishbein's words, that there was "a small percentage of doctors who could not be trusted in this respect."

Meanwhile, of course, the country was mired in the Great Depression, and President Roosevelt was about to launch his New Deal. The AMA's president-elect in 1933, Dean Lewis, MD, expressed the view that the medical profession had performed admirably during this type of adversity.

"In some ways," he told the delegates, "the Depression has rendered a great service, as it has been demonstrated that many of the mechanical aids to practice are not necessary and that the cost of medical service may be greatly reduced…Simplification of medical practice should be the aim of this organization. Such simplification will mean a limitation of specialism and the reduction of specialists."

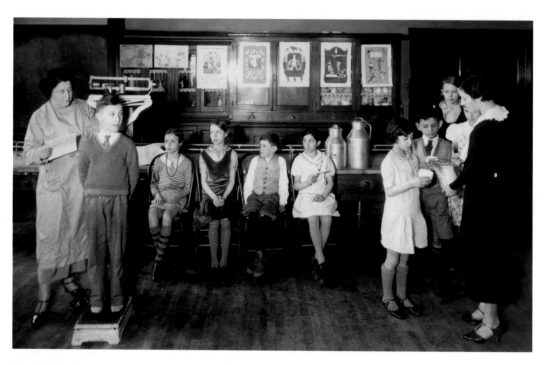

The Chicago Woman's Aid Society sponsored a free milk program for children in 1915.

The Depression brings renewed controversy over medical benefits legislation

Despite Dr Lewis' brave words, the Depression had a profound effect on physicians and patients alike. The AMA went on record encouraging county medical societies to share the burden of caring for needy patients. Countless physicians provided untold thousands of hours of free care or took their payment in farm produce, services, or other barterable items. But as conditions worsened, advocates of various national health schemes

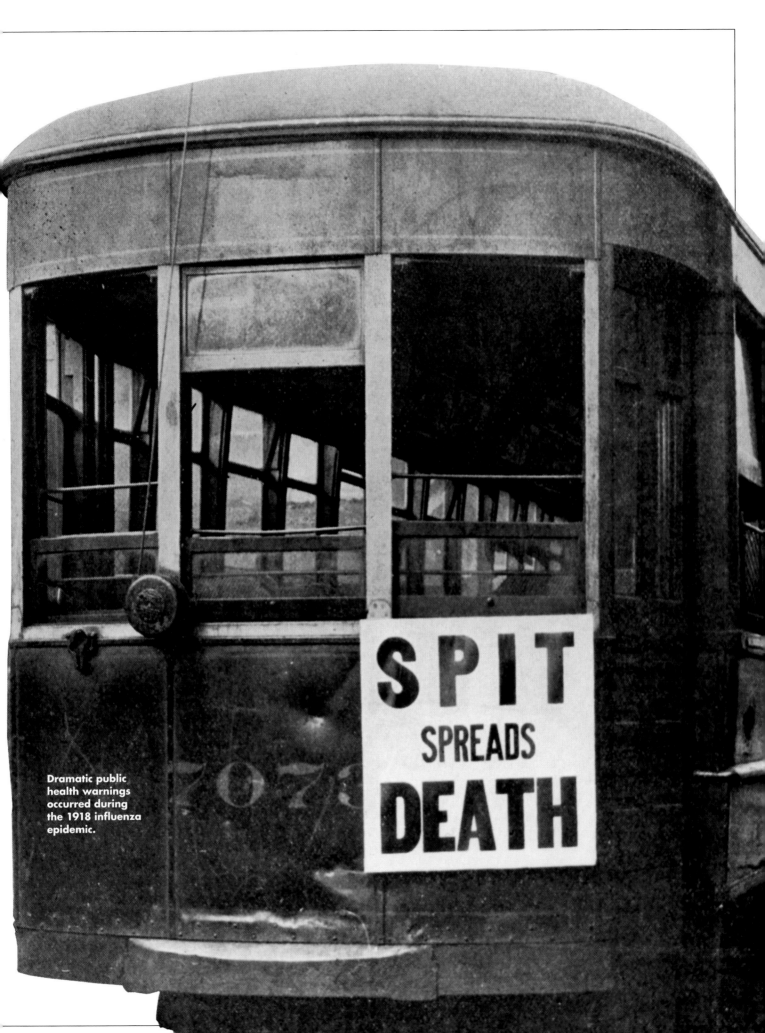

Dramatic public health warnings occurred during the 1918 influenza epidemic.

SPIT
SPREADS
DEATH

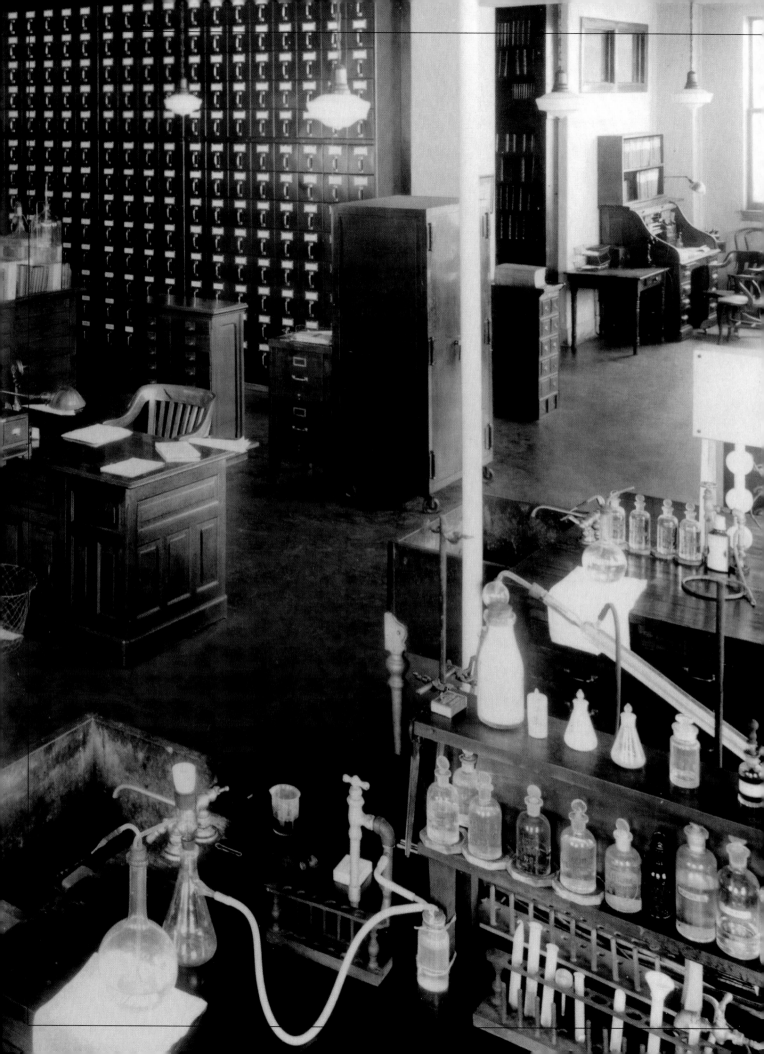

were quick to point to their ideas as potential remedies, and the government's role was expanding steadily. The AMA Judicial Council, commenting on the activities of the Emergency Relief Administration, stated in 1934: "One of the strongest holds of the profession on public approbation and support has been the age-old professional ideal of medical service to all, whether able to pay or not…The abandonment of that ideal and the adoption of a principle of service only when paid for would be the greatest step toward socialized medicine and shortly state medicine which the medical profession could take."

In 1935, the Democratic Administration launched a legislative trial balloon that would have included substantial medical benefits in the original Social Security bill. President Roosevelt was unwilling to make this a major issue in the face of certain opposition from the AMA, and the idea was abandoned. The AMA's cause was greatly helped by the efforts of Harvey Cushing, MD, the noted surgeon and educator and one of the most admired members of the profession. He held no AMA office, but he was a strong ally — and his daughter was married to President Roosevelt's oldest son, James. Dr Cushing was appointed to an advisory committee to the Committee on Economic Security, where he expressed his views against government medicine. As things turned out, the Social Security Act included only a few provisions for medical care — provisions for infant and maternal health and aid for the crippled and blind — that were acceptable to medicine.

By 1938, as the Depression lingered, the issue of medical benefits resurfaced. Responding to a federally initiated National Health Conference, the AMA House of Delegates met in special session and endorsed voluntary, prepaid, hospital service insurance (which later became Blue Cross). As this was going on, the AMA had received warnings that the US Department of Justice was preparing an indictment of the AMA as a monopoly. That indictment, naming also the Medical Society of the District of Columbia, the Harris County (Texas) Medical Society, and various individuals, was

The Mayo Clinic's Charles Mayo, MD, was summoned to San Francisco when President Warren G. Harding developed pneumonia.

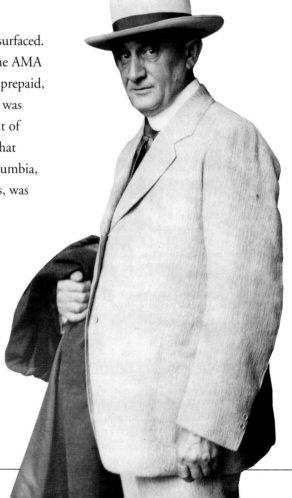

Facing page: Before World War II, the AMA established its own chemical laboratory to evaluate drugs.

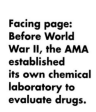

brought before a grand jury in 1938, and a criminal indictment was returned in 1939. The defendants were charged with denying hospital privileges to physicians associated with the Group Health Association of Washington, a prepaid plan, by withholding membership in local medical societies. The case, brought under the Sherman Antitrust Act, would continue in court for some 4 years.

World War II and new medical advancements

As the 1930s wound down, the AMA was preparing and mounting its defense against the antitrust charges, and the pace of world events was accelerating. The Depression was ending, but war was looming. Military preparedness was an issue, and the military surgeon general had already contacted the AMA to ensure assistance in the mobilization of physicians. Congress had just adopted the Food, Drug and Cosmetic Act. The influx of refugee physicians from Europe was increasing. Senator Robert Wagner of New York had introduced a national health bill in New York that would stimulate hotly debated legislation in the coming decade (Roosevelt initially supported it, then backed away), and discussions of socialized medicine were pushing ahead in England.

This physician (below, at right) was employed by a Texas farm project to provide care to families working on the project.

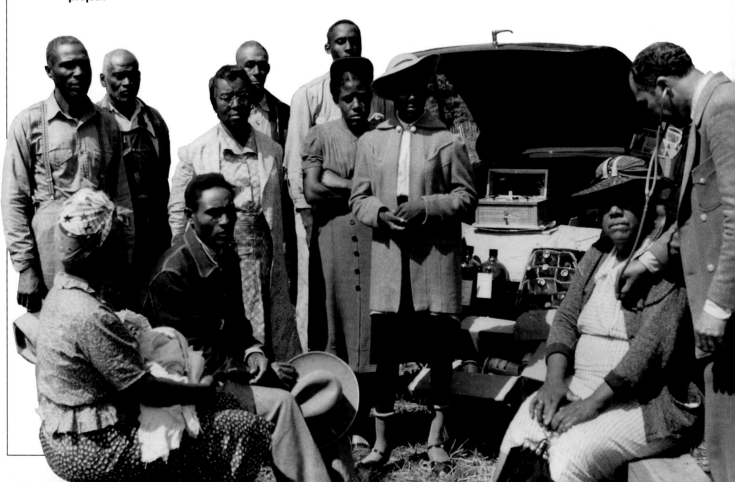

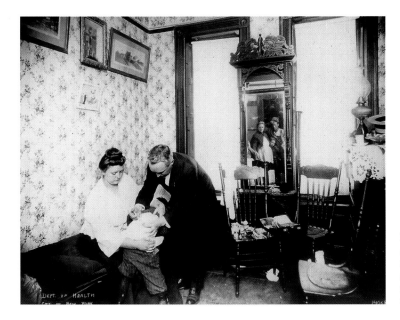

House calls were commonplace; at left, a physician administers diphtheria antitoxin as family members watch and wait.

Meanwhile, scientific developments in the 1930s would usher in one of medicine's most exciting eras. In 1935, a German biochemist, Gerhard Domagk, who was working on dyes, discovered that Prontosil could cure streptococcal infections in mice. In one of the serendipitous developments that seem to fill medical history books, Domagk's young daughter was suffering from a streptococcal disease that was not responding to conventional therapy, so he administered Prontosil. Her immediate and complete recovery stimulated more research; it turned out that the human body metabolized Prontosil into sulfanilamide — the first of the "magic bullet" drugs.

Even more dramatic was British physician Alexander Fleming's earlier accidental discovery of a germicidal fungus that he identified as *Penicillium notatum* and that directly attacked staphylococci. Because Fleming's hospital lacked the resources for further research, development of this discovery was eventually pursued by two other scientists. They shared the Nobel Prize with Fleming, who was later knighted, and by the time World War II ended, enough penicillin was being produced to serve the needs of the military and the civilian populations alike.

The early years of the 20th century had seen major, dramatic developments in the science of medicine. One of the American Medical Association's prime accomplishments in that period was its role in elevating the quality of medical education, ensuring that this new explosion of knowledge would reach qualified students and physicians.

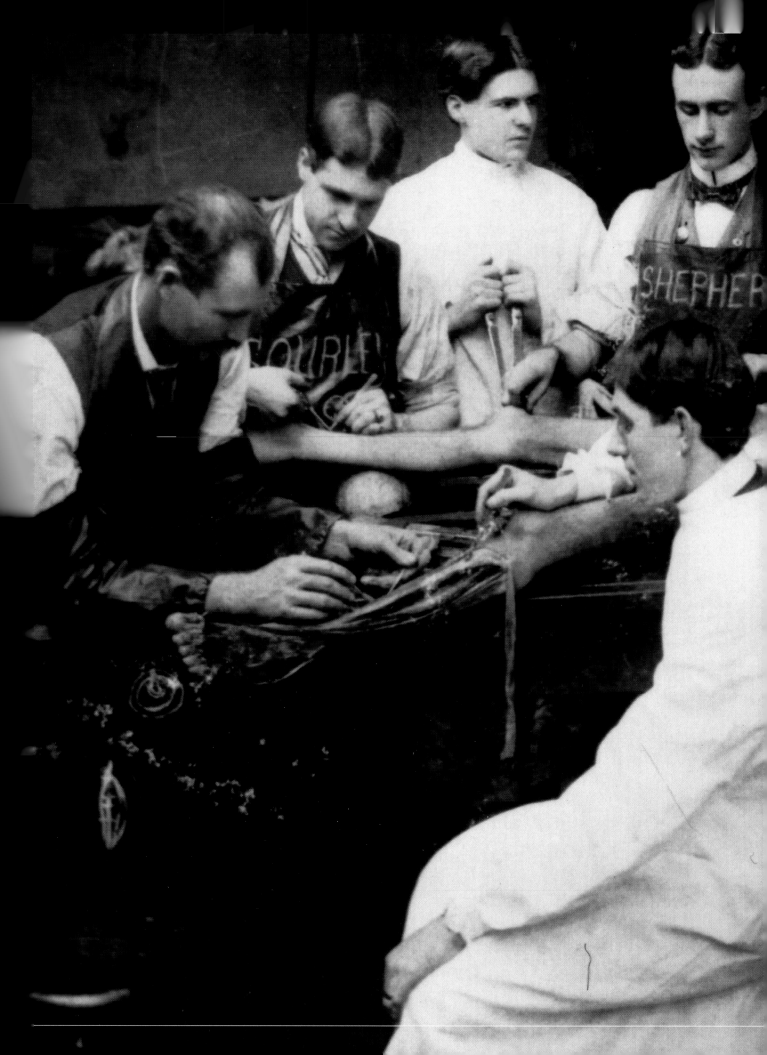

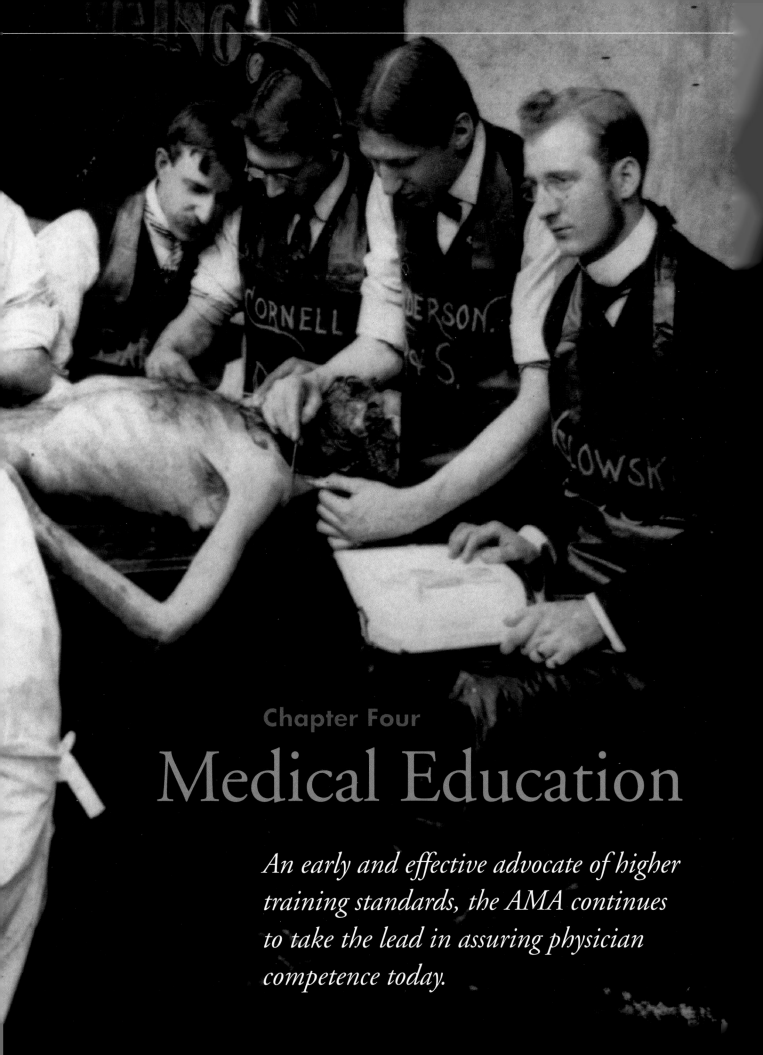

Chapter Four

Medical Education

An early and effective advocate of higher training standards, the AMA continues to take the lead in assuring physician competence today.

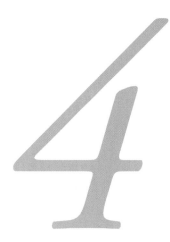

Medical Education

Although improving the quality of medical education had been one of the stated goals of the founders of the American Medical Association, the organization's impact did not begin to be felt in a major way until the beginning of the 20th century.

This was not because of a lack of effort on the AMA's part. Founder Nathan S. Davis, MD, among many others, labored tirelessly to convince medical schools to upgrade their standards, but the impact was limited. Although some institutions greatly upgraded their entrance and graduation requirements and broadened their curriculums to keep pace with the scientific advances that were taking place, many of the so-called diploma mills remained in existence for decades.

Just after the turn of the century, however, a series of significant and related events occurred. The AMA and others had noted that only a few medical schools required students to have any college education before enrolling; a few did not require a high school diploma. However, the growing stature of the AMA, the advances in science and medical technology, and the public's growing interest in the qualifications of caregivers combined to create a climate in which reforms could thrive.

In 1904, the American Medical Association created its Council on Medical Education, giving it the assignment of accelerating organized medicine's

Overleaf: Students in the anatomy lab in 1905 at the College of Physicians & Surgeons of Illinois, later the University of Illinois Medical School.

efforts to raise the educational requirements for physicians. The Council wasted little time. In 1905, the Council, relying largely on a curriculum developed at The Johns Hopkins University School of Medicine in Baltimore, published far-reaching statements outlining the minimum and ideal standards for a medical school. A well-educated physician, the Council said, should meet these ideals:

- **undergraduate study of the basic sciences of biology, chemistry, and physics;**

- **2 years of medical school training in the laboratory sciences, including anatomy, physiology, microbiology, pathology, and pharmacology;**

- **2 more years of medical school training in clinical medicine, including surgery, internal medicine, pediatrics, obstetrics, and others; this training, the Council emphasized, should take place "in close contact with patients in dispensaries and hospitals"; and**

- **a year of graduate education in a hospital, the precursor of the formalized internship program.**

A year later, the Council on Medical Education took another major step, publishing the first complete directory of medical schools in the United States, including details on the admissions requirements. At this point, only five of the 160 medical schools listed in the directory required any college-level training in the biological and physical sciences. Also published in *JAMA* was information from state licensing boards identifying medical schools whose graduates had the highest failure rates on their licensing examinations.

The Council on Medical Education continued its relentless drive for improvements. A tour of the 162 medical schools that existed during 1906–1907 was undertaken by various members of the Council, frequently in the company of the Council's secretary, the indefatigable Nathan P. Colwell, MD.

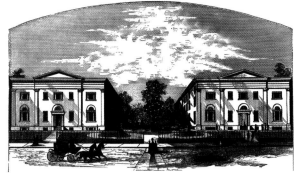

UNIVERSITY OF PENNSYLVANIA.

The University of Pennsylvania School of Medicine as it looked in 1850.

In 1907 came another major offensive: the Council compiled a 10-point standard of medical school inspection, calling for scrutiny of laboratory facilities and instruction, dispensary facilities and training, and hospital facilities and instruction. At the same time, the Council was appointing a committee of 100 physicians to look at the entire medical school curriculum.

The Flexner Report

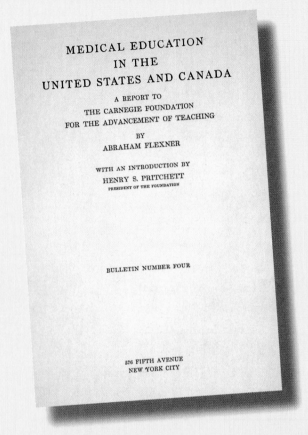

MEDICAL EDUCATION
IN THE
UNITED STATES AND CANADA

A REPORT TO
THE CARNEGIE FOUNDATION
FOR THE ADVANCEMENT OF TEACHING

BY
ABRAHAM FLEXNER

WITH AN INTRODUCTION BY
HENRY S. PRITCHETT
PRESIDENT OF THE FOUNDATION

BULLETIN NUMBER FOUR

576 FIFTH AVENUE
NEW YORK CITY

The Flexner report is widely hailed as the first major step in reforming the medical education system in this country. It minced no words and spared no sensibilities. Written in terms that would raise the pulse rate of many lawyers today, its impact was immediate and widespread. Some examples of the straightforward language are shown below.

Referring to a school in Chattanooga:
"This is a typical example of the schools that claim to exist for the sake of the poor boy and the back country."

Further north:
"Wisconsin presents a simple problem: the two Milwaukee schools are without a redeeming feature."

And in the AMA's home town, with 14 medical schools at the time:
"The city of Chicago is in respect to medical education the plague spot of the country."

Flexner noted that Illinois state laws and requirements were adequate to mandate quality instruction; however,
"With the indubitable connivance of the state board, these provisions are, and have been, flagrantly violated."

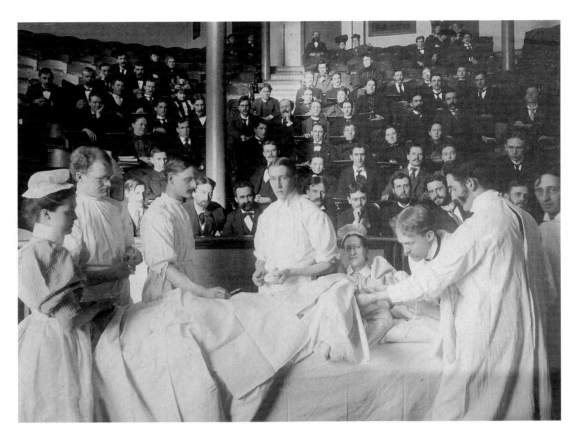

The surgical
clinic at Chicago's
Northwestern
Medical School
around the turn
of the century.
Student nurses
from Wesley
Hospital are
assisting.

In 1909, that body's report was adopted. It described a 4,000-hour medical school curriculum designed to serve as a model for any school wishing to revise its curriculum.

In 1910, the Council moved ahead again, publishing the first "Essentials of an Acceptable Medical College." The statement covered 25 key areas, dealing with such areas as faculty qualifications, library facilities, grading policies, record keeping, attendance, and admissions. A significant passage recommended that the medical school own or control a hospital, enabling students to have "close and extended contact with patients under the supervision of the attending staff."

The Flexner Report: a watershed event in medical education

The publication of the Essentials was a major milestone with long-term implications; the AMA would revise the Essentials several times before supplanting them in 1957 with the "Functions and Structure of a Medical School." But the watershed event in medical education in 1910 was the publication of the Flexner Report. This far-reaching activity, funded by the Carnegie Foundation for the Advancement of Teaching and supported enthusiastically by the AMA, took the foundation's Abraham Flexner and the AMA's Dr Colwell on another tour of the 131 medical schools then

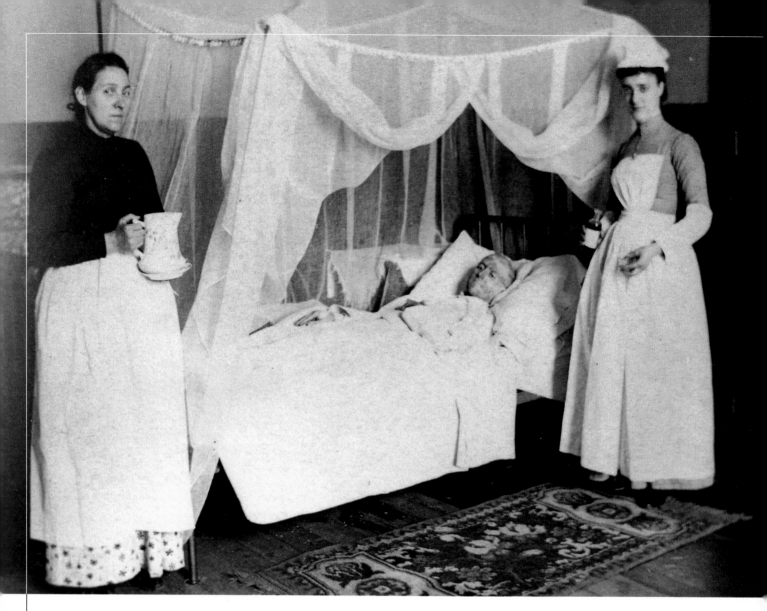

Residency training has always been accompanied by the risk of contracting communicable diseases from patients. James W. Pelham, MD, a resident at Philadelphia General Hospital, was recovering from tuberculosis in 1888.

doing business in the United States. The eight Canadian medical schools also asked to be surveyed, so they were included as well.

The Flexner report also expressed concern for the students and future students, expressing "a hearty sympathy for the American youth who, too often the prey of commercial advertising methods, is steered into the practice of medicine with almost no opportunity to learn the difference between an efficient medical school and a hopelessly inadequate one. A clerk who is receiving $50 a month in the country store gets an alluring brochure which paints the life of the physician as an easy road to wealth. He has no realization of the difference between medicine as a profession and medicine as a business…."

Flexner also addressed the issue of women physicians, noting that while more schools were opening their doors to women students, "fewer attend and fewer graduate." He questioned the need for separate schools and hospitals for women, but added that if these were not developed, "interne [sic] privileges must be granted to women graduates on the same terms as men."

Flexner's report presented the concerns of the public as well, concluding that the "interests of the general public have been so generally lost sight of in this matter that the public has in large measure forgot that it has any interests to protect. And yet in no other way does education more closely touch the individual than in the quality of medical training…."

After the Flexner report the AMA focused new attention *on graduate training.*

The Flexner report sounded the death knell for the diploma mills. The next pivotal step was the founding in 1912 of the Federation of State Medical Boards, which agreed to accept the AMA's evaluation of medical schools as authoritative.

The Council on Medical Education then turned its focus to postgraduate training, developing the first standards for approved internships and publishing in 1914 the first list of hospitals whose internship programs complied with those standards. The first formal "Essentials of Approved Internships" was published in 1919, and a year later the Council's name was changed to Council on Medical Education and Hospitals to reflect the broadened responsibilities. (The Council reverted to its original name in 1963.)

Pre-med students in the laboratory at the University of Illinois.

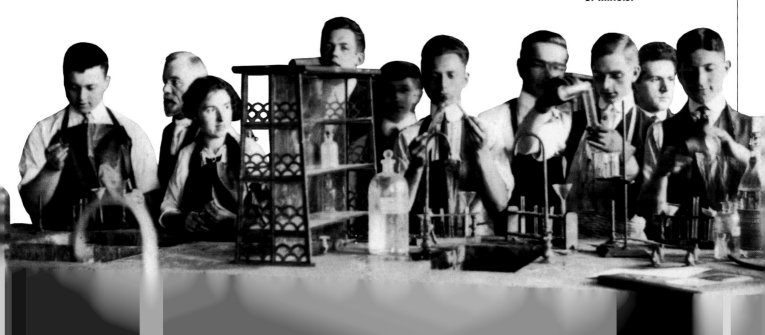

The AMA's continuing role in medical education

The American Medical Association's role in medical education has continued undiminished since the early part of the century. Today, the AMA is an active participant in establishing training standards at every level. The Council on Medical Education's site inspections continued until 1942, when the AMA and the Association of American Medical Colleges (AAMC) joined to form the Liaison Committee on Medical Education to conduct accreditation programs on a joint basis. A decade later, the US Department of Organization received the blessing of the federal government to designate approved medical schools at which returning World War II veterans could use their GI bill benefits. The Department of Health, Education, and Welfare in 1968 certified the Liaison Committee on Medical Education as the official accrediting agency for undergraduate medical education. The membership of this committee now includes representatives of the AMA, the AAMC, the Committee on Accreditation of Canadian Medical Schools, and two public members.

Beyond the undergraduate medical education level, the AMA continues to have a strong presence. As the movement to graduate training leading to specialization gathered steam in the early part of the century, the AMA Council on Medical Education became a force. A landmark 1920 report found a great demand for specialty training, but a lack of adequate facilities — a gap that should not be met by proprietary institutions, the Council said: "It would be desirable for 15 to 20 strong university medical departments to consider the development of graduate medical departments." The Council then appointed committees to recommend courses of training in 15 specialties: internal medicine, pediatrics, neuropsychiatry, orthopedic surgery, dermatology and syphilology, surgery, ophthalmology, otolaryngology, urology, obstetrics and gynecology, public health and hygiene, anatomy, physiology, pharmacology and therapeutics, and pathology-bacteriology.

In 1923, the Council published "Principles Regarding Graduate Medical Education" and 4 years later issued the first listing of hospitals approved for residency training. The "Essentials of Approved Residencies" then appeared in 1928. Developing a cooperative arrangement for accrediting residency programs would not be as easy as uniting the profession to upgrade undergraduate education, however, because of the diversity of the organizations legitimately involved.

It was, in fact, not until 1972 that accord was reached among the major players in postgraduate education that led to the formation of the Liaison Committee on Graduate Medical Education, which became the Accreditation

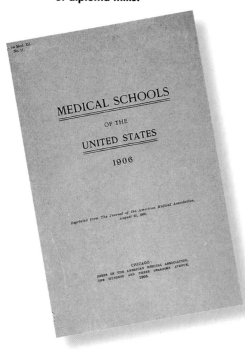

AMA's first directory of medical schools, published in 1906, was a major step toward the demise of diploma mills.

*The growth of specialties
posed new challenges;*
**the AMA took the
lead in advocating
university training.**

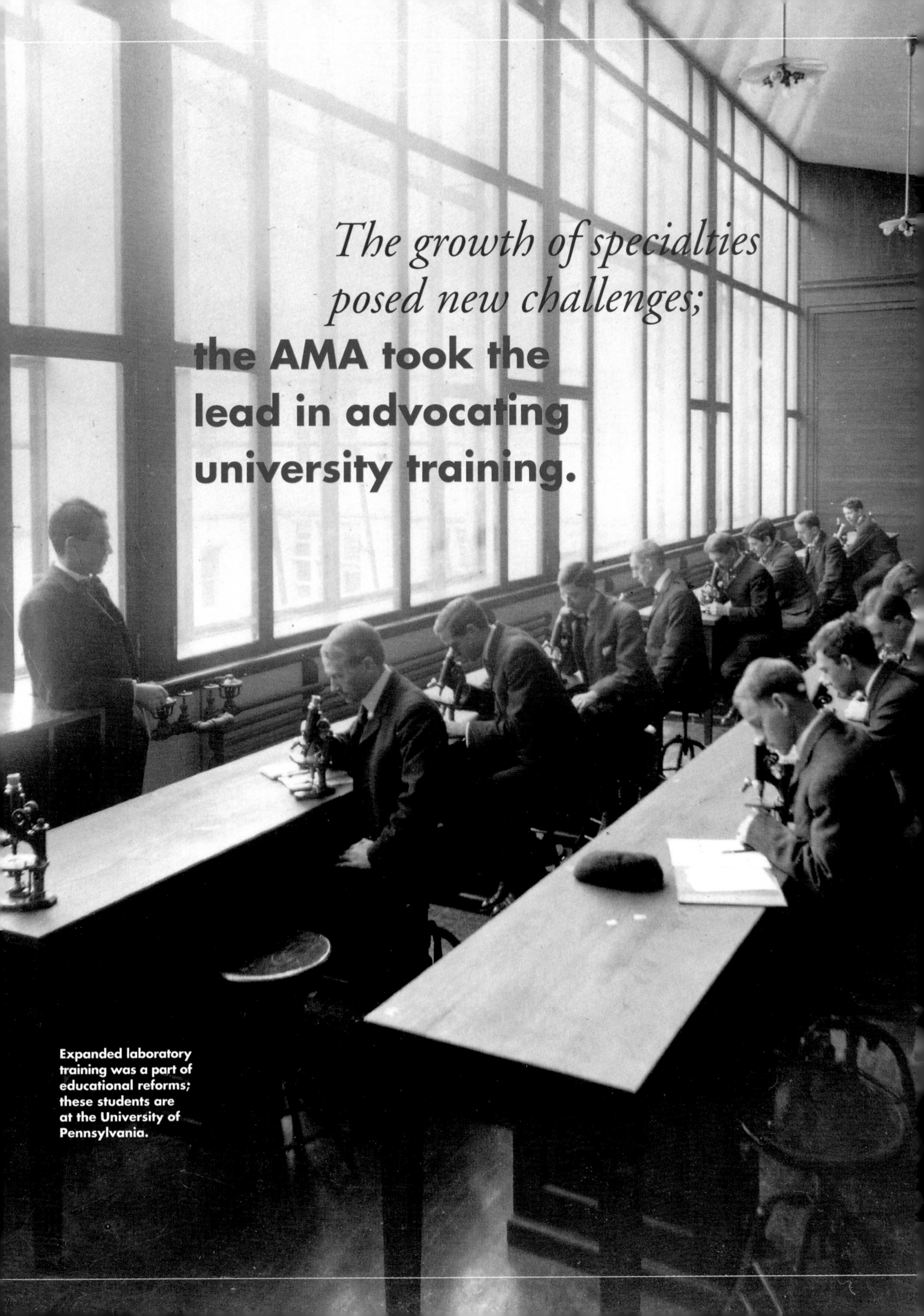

Expanded laboratory
training was a part of
educational reforms;
these students are
at the University of
Pennsylvania.

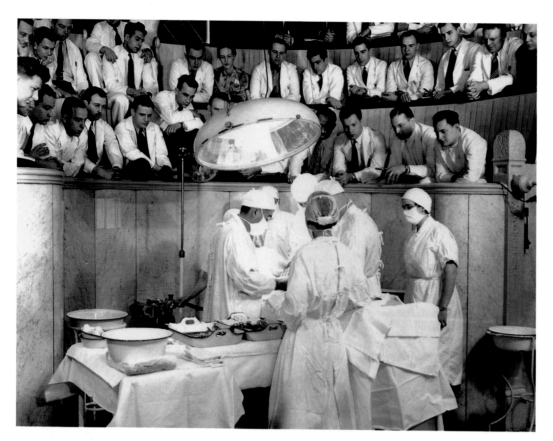

Students at Chicago's Rush Medical College watch Fred O. Priest, MD, perform surgery in 1938.

Council for Graduate Medical Education. After intense negotiations and debate, membership slots on this new body were allocated among the American Medical Association, Association of American Medical Colleges, American Board of Medical Specialties, Council of Medical Specialty Societies, and American Hospital Association. Seats for a federal government representative, a public representative, and a resident physician representative were also included.

The next step was the continuing education of physicians — a minor issue in the early part of the century but, with the explosion in technology, a major component in the assurance of high-quality care. The Accreditation Council for Continuing Medical Education, with membership from the AMA and other organizations involved in continuing medical education, is the major player in this burgeoning industry. The AMA also publishes a *Directory of Continuing Medical Education* and, since 1968, has presented the Physician's Recognition Award to those physicians who meet specific continuing education guidelines.

Today, the Council on Medical Education's activities continue to reflect current trends and problems confronting the profession. Physician workforce issues — determining what constitutes an adequate supply of physicians and making sure that the needs of the public are being met — is an ongoing issue. Generations of physicians in this country have completed their training and gone forth into their chosen field, relatively confident of the future. Today, however, changing market forces and the inexorable push toward some variation of managed care have clouded the outlook for those trained in some fields. Such high-tech developments as telemedicine further complicate the picture, and the explosion of clinical knowledge is forcing constant reevaluation of the curriculum.

An ongoing commitment to quality medical education

Throughout the continuum of medical education, medical students and physicians in the United States are never very far from the influence of the American Medical Association. On the surface, the impact is barely apparent; it is there nonetheless. The prospective medical student, eyeing the admissions requirements for the school of his/her choice, will find in place undergraduate training requisites that stem directly from the AMA's activities nearly a century ago. The AMA does not set these standards, of course, but the early impact of the Council on Medical Education is still felt.

This influence goes on throughout the 4 years of medical school — remember the "Essentials of an Approved Medical College" back in 1910 — through the residency period (the "Essentials of an Approved Residency"), and through whatever continuing education courses the physician may choose to undertake. In fact, a convincing argument can be made that the American Medical Association's most significant contribution to raising the standards of medical care in this country to the level of excellence it has enjoyed for many years has been its willingness to involve itself in the difficult issues surrounding medical education.

None of this has been done alone, of course. The entire medical profession — particularly medical specialty societies and the education community — can take credit. There is probably no profession anywhere whose members have been so willing to commit as much time and energy as physicians have done for the good of the profession and their patients. And there is probably no other profession whose various professional organizations have been willing to set aside differences in philosophy and personality to work together to develop, implement, and monitor standards of excellence for their members and future members. The credit for much of this progress should be shared across the profession. However, the leadership role has, for the most part, been borne by the American Medical Association.

Organized medicine continues to **work tirelessly to develop and monitor high standards** *for all levels of training.*

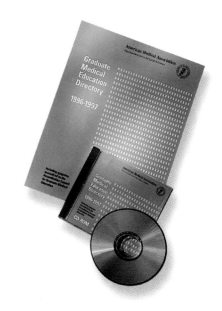

To respond to changes in how people access information, AMA published its reference work, *Graduate Medical Education Directory,* as a book and also as a CD-ROM.

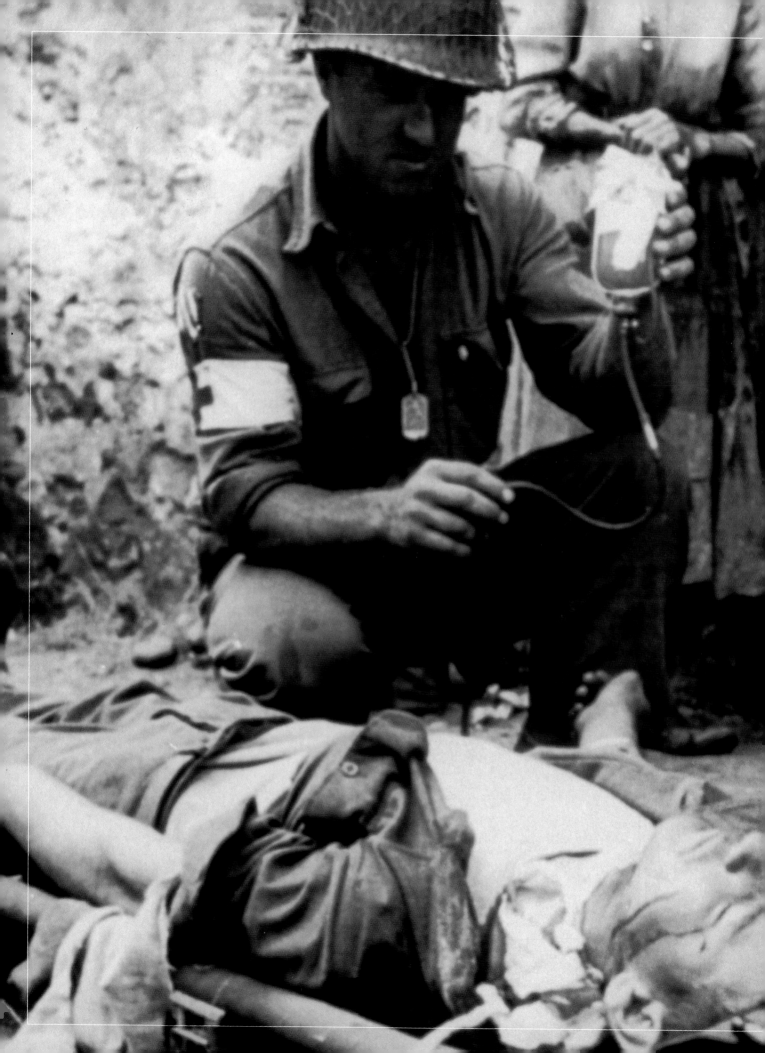

1940 to 1950

World War II dominated this turbulent decade and had a long-term effect on many facets of medicine.

5

1940 to 1950

As the 1940s began, war was on the horizon. The coming conflict would dramatically reshape the world order. For medicine, the lives of thousands of physicians would be altered irrevocably. Beyond that, World War II would be instrumental in several dramatic scientific advances and would have profound implications on the way medical care was delivered.

In 1940, the AMA met in New York City. The president, Wisconsin psychiatrist Rock Sleyster, MD, spoke of the need for preparedness. He recalled the involvement of the AMA in obtaining medical personnel in World War I and stated: "Today our nation is again preparing to defend itself to the utmost against any type of aggression from without. The medical profession, through its House of Delegates, I know, will pledge itself to give, as it has always given in the past, every iota of service that it is capable of rendering."

The House of Delegates was quick to respond, pledging "unstinting support of the federal government in the campaign for preparedness in the present chaotic state of a world in which right and reason have been cast to the winds and only brute force is recognized and heeded." The House also authorized appointment of a Committee on Medical Preparedness. Also, the National Research Council had asked the AMA to launch a periodical covering research and military medicine; this became the journal *War Medicine*.

Overleaf: A wounded US soldier receives plasma in Sicily during the Allies' invasion.

Hanging over the future of the Association was the antitrust suit filed in 1939, charging violations of the Sherman Act. The Supreme Court had denied the petition of the AMA and its codefendants, making a trial in US District Court inevitable, and the AMA and all the defendants were ordered to be in Washington on June 14, 1940, to appear before the court. The Board of Trustees authorized a plea of not guilty.

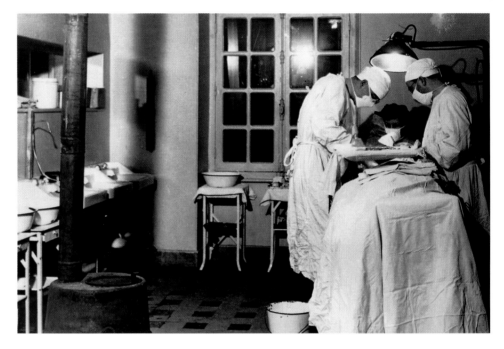

US military surgeons in action at the 27th Evacuation Hospital in Darmstadt, Germany.

In April 1941, the district court jury in Washington found all of the individual defendants in the antitrust case not guilty, but the AMA and the Medical Society of the District of Columbia were found guilty and fined $2500 and $1500, respectively. A final appeal was denied by the Supreme Court in 1943.

The same two issues — war and litigation — continued to occupy center stage as the attack on Pearl Harbor drew nearer.

One effect of World War II on the medical community would have been easy to predict. Thousands of physicians entered the military. They served all over the globe, on ships, in trenches, in high-tech hospitals, in basic training facilities — wherever there was an American military presence, medical care was available. These physicians sacrificed years of their careers, at great personal risk. In return, they received commissions and assignments that ranged from daily confrontations with combat and danger to the tedium of taking sick call — and conducting venereal disease inspections — in basic training installations.

The good news was that battlefield medicine during World War II for the first time was saving lives through up-to-date scientific techniques. For the first time in a war, shock was warded off by administration of plasma. Medics could administer syrettes of morphine. Wounds were cleaned with iodine and packed with antibacterial powders such as sulfanilamide, with penicillin becoming widely available as the war wore on. The first true antibiotics were available. In addition, US troops in World War II were better fed than in any previous conflict. Immunizations and improved sanitation virtually eliminated some of the major causes of death in earlier wars — diphtheria, typhoid, cholera, dysentery, and smallpox.

For the doctors who stayed at home — by and large the older physicians, those with medical problems of their own, and women — the burdens were great also. Many came out of retirement when the call to arms left their communities short of physicians. All worked long hours without adequate backup; many would go months at a time without a day off.

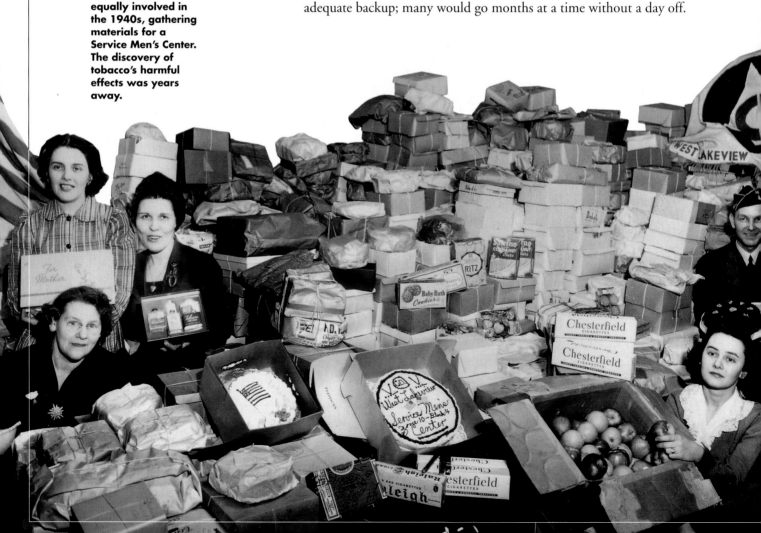

The home front was equally involved in the 1940s, gathering materials for a Service Men's Center. The discovery of tobacco's harmful effects was years away.

The rise of medical specialization

The war also had a long-term impact on medical specialization and training that would have been difficult to foresee. When a physician went into the military service during World War II, the difference between a specialist and a generalist became immediately apparent. The physician who could demonstrate some background of specialty training — 2 years of a residency would do — received a commission as an Army or Air Force captain (or a Navy lieutenant). Those without specialty training came in one grade lower — as first lieutenants in the Army and Air Force, or as a lieutenant junior grade in the Navy.

This, of course, meant some slight differential in pay and status; more important were the duty assignments that followed. In the military hierarchy, the upper ranks and many of the choice assignments were the province of the specialist. For the generalist, military duty was summed up by the AMA's Richard Egan, MD, a long-time educator: "Soon he is overseas with a tactical unit. As a battalion surgeon, he has to see that the kitchen is clean, inspect the latrines, do the short-arm inspections, and in combat tend the wounded under fire and sleep in a wet foxhole. He probably is a captain by now. But his friends are majors and lieutenant colonels. And they're back in Paris, Honolulu, London, or Walter Reed doing interesting things in the advanced technology of military hospitals. [The generalist] considers himself, at times, just a high-paid aid man."

Another catalyst toward the rush to specialization was the passage in Congress of the Serviceman's Readjustment Act of 1944, better known to this day as the GI Bill of Rights. It included postgraduate medical education, opening the door for thousands of returning military physicians to all sorts of advanced activities. As physicians returned from the war, the prospect of federally subsidized graduate training loomed invitingly. Additionally, military service provided physicians a new look at many practice and lifestyle options. To many, the life of a small-town generalist in solo practice (and on call around the clock) didn't seem quite so appealing.

The 24-hours-on-call life also had lost much of its appeal for the physicians who didn't go to war. In 1943–1944, about a third of the physician population was serving in the military, leading to enormous pressures on those left behind. As the war wound down, they too envisioned a life that might include time for an occasional movie or concert as well as a practice with a partner or partners with whom on-call status might be shared. For some, a specialty residency seemed to be a highly desirable step in that direction.

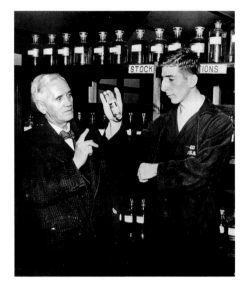

Sir Alexander Fleming (left), who pioneered the use of penicillin, visits with a wounded soldier at the 15th US Army Hospital who had been successfully treated with the drug.

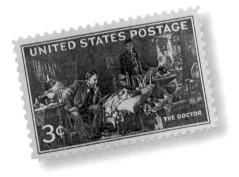

Honoring AMA's centennial, the US Postal Service issued a commemorative stamp featuring a famous painting by Sir Luke Fildes.

Another piece of wartime legislation also had major long-term effects. The Public Health Service Act of 1944 put the federal government into biomedical research in a big way. The first National Institutes of Health grants in 1945 totaled $85,000. They mushroomed to $850,000 in 1946 and to $8.5 million by 1950 — a substantial sum at that time. Most of the money went to medical schools or to scientists doing research in medical schools. This funding paved the way for the research that produced many of the breakthroughs that followed — organ transplantation, heart-lung machines, and entire new generations of drugs. And as medical science advanced by quantum leaps, the move toward specialization became unstoppable.

After the war, increased funding nourished the growth of science and research.

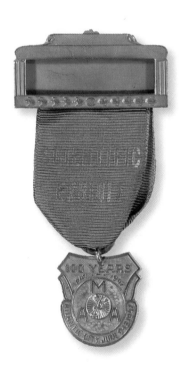

An AMA delegate's centennial badge from 1947.

Of all the factors that launched the boom in specialization that got under way in the 1940s and would continue for most of the remainder of the century, the most significant was the explosion in scientific knowledge. Medicine was becoming so complex that it became unrealistic to expect any one individual to be totally competent in all its facets. And as specialists devoted full time to a particular area of study, the body of knowledge about that topic could only expand.

Wartime and postwar changes for AMA

By war's end, the AMA also had undergone some major changes. The Association had thrown itself wholeheartedly into the war effort, devoting major resources and staff time to meeting requests of government agencies that began with the military but also covered large sectors of the home front. A 1943 report of the Board of Trustees detailed some of the activities, stating that "Members of all of the Councils, the members of the Board of Trustees and the administrative personnel in practically every department have served in various capacities on committees or commissions of official standing in Washington or in other ways have...devoted a large part of their time to such service. Official representatives of the Association have on numerous occasions been called on to participate in official conferences held in Washington and have attempted in that connection and in many other ways to be as helpful as possible to the federal government."

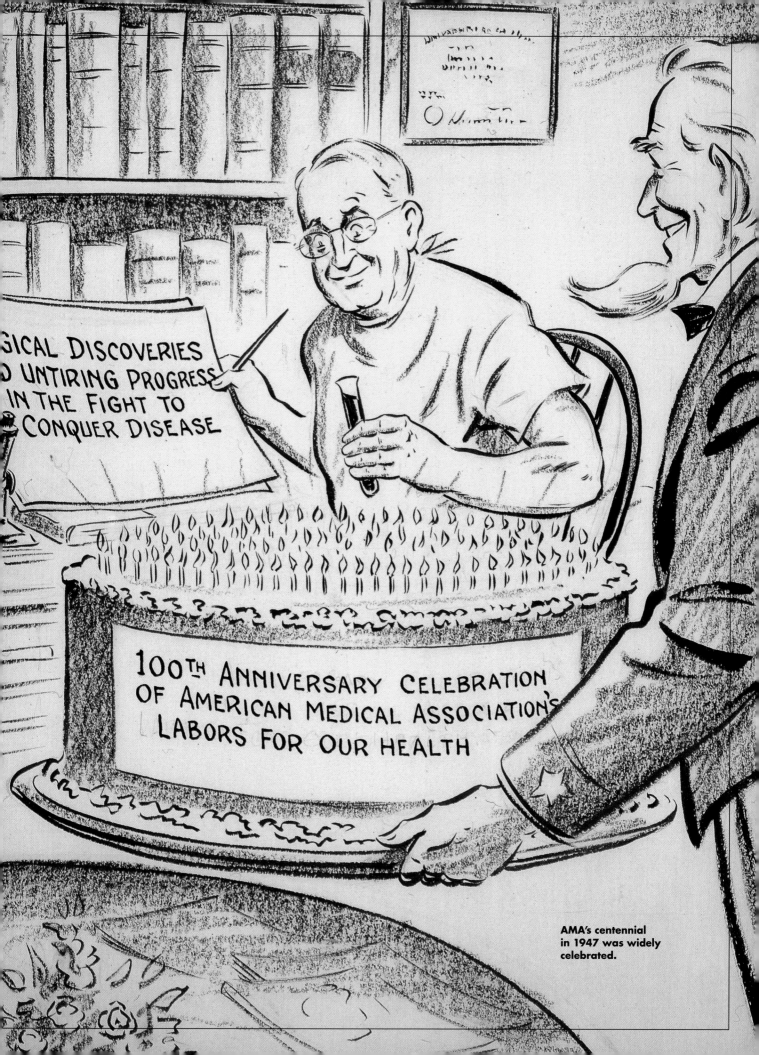

GICAL DISCOVERIES
D UNTIRING PROGRESS
IN THE FIGHT TO
CONQUER DISEASE

100TH ANNIVERSARY CELEBRATION
OF AMERICAN MEDICAL ASSOCIATION'S
LABORS FOR OUR HEALTH

AMA's centennial
in 1947 was widely
celebrated.

The AMA also was looking beyond the war. By 1943, the Council on Medical Education and Hospitals was studying the specialty certification issue. The Association's president, Fred W. Rankin, MD, was serving as a brigadier general in charge of surgical services in the Office of the Surgeon General of the Army. In his address to the AMA House of Delegates, he

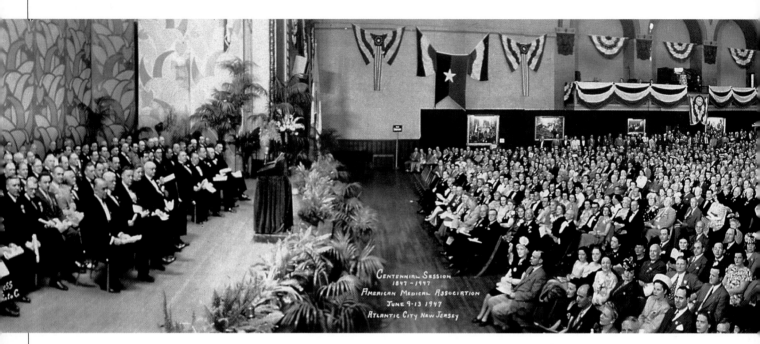

CENTENNIAL SESSION
1847-1947
AMERICAN MEDICAL ASSOCIATION
JUNE 9-13 1947
ATLANTIC CITY NEW JERSEY

made note of the wartime problems but also considered the societal changes that were altering the way medicine was being practiced. These had been developing over time, he said, warning: "We must face realistically these tremendous socioeconomic trends."

Despite the urgencies of the war, the AMA in 1943 was at a crossroads regarding its future: should it devote itself totally to scientific activities, or should it involve itself in what was certain to be a major public debate over the financing of medical care? The AMA's secretary/general manager, Olin West, MD, citing fears of possible government retribution, argued strongly against political activism. But at its 1943 meeting, the House of Delegates authorized a Washington office. Even more importantly, the delegates established a powerful new body, the Council on Medical Service and Public Relations, and gave it specific nonscientific objectives. In doing so, it created a major new arm of the organization — reporting directly to the House of Delegates, not the Board of Trustees — that would go on to play a major role in the battle over national health care legislation in the 1940s and 1950s.

Dr Fishbein remained firmly in charge throughout the war years, however, and in 1944 he summed up some of the AMA's major activities in the war effort. He pointed out that the AMA was aiding in the training in physical

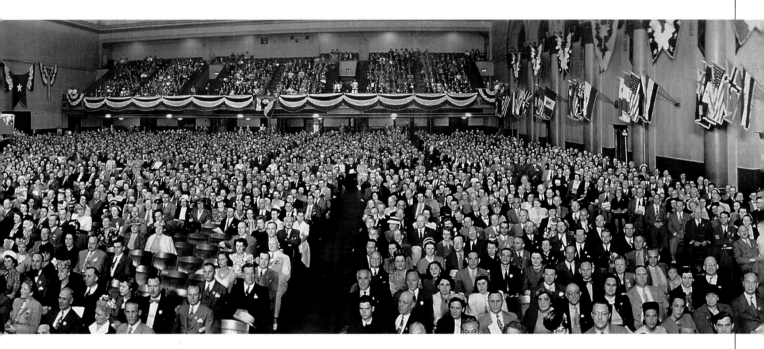

A panoramic view of AMA's centennial meeting in 1947 in Atlantic City, NJ.

therapy; the Committee on Postwar Medical Service was considering graduate training for physicians returning from the military. Some 18,000 copies of *JAMA* were being sent to physicians serving overseas in various branches of the armed forces. AMA officers and staff were involved with the National Research Council in developing lists of essential drugs and of standards for the control and distribution of food.

Ironically, the importance of radio as a communications medium would soon diminish. In 1946, with television a relative infant, the AMA began television broadcasts of health messages to the general public. At the same time, the AMA was providing dramatic programming on two major radio networks — the National Broadcasting Chain and the Mutual Broadcasting Chain — and was distributing specially prepared recorded messages on health that were in widespread usage by many individual stations. The year 1946 also saw the formation of a new department of public relations at AMA headquarters. The department was preparing a weekly bulletin to the press on scientific advances (this is still done today), a letter to the

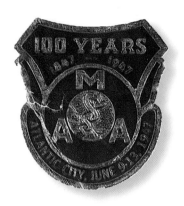

An AMA centennial seal, 1947.

headquarters of state and county medical societies, and general publicity work for the organization.

Centennial celebration: summing up and looking forward

The end of the war meant a time for some reevaluation of Association goals and priorities. First, however, it meant plans for a major observance of the AMA's 100th birthday. One important event was the publication of Dr Fishbein's epic *History of the American Medical Association 1847 to 1947.* The US Postal Service issued a special commemorative stamp. The AMA's secretary, George F. Lull, MD, reported that 5389 new members had been added during the previous 12 months, making a total membership of 132,224 as of April 1, 1947 — a record.

The annual meeting was held that year in Atlantic City, NJ. The Association's president, Harrison H. Shoulders, MD, of Nashville, discussing the organization's first 100 years, stated:

"[t]he changes which have taken place in the knowledge, technics and tools of medicine have not brought about a change in the philosophy of medicine… There has been no need for change. The philosophy of medicine has been, and still is, a philosophy of progress, a progress which is restricted only by prudence and caution…It is a philosophy of service. It places service to humanity above all other considerations. It is a philosophy of freedom. It recognizes the dignity and importance of human individuality and that it is in an atmosphere of freedom that this individuality finds opportunity for its highest forms of expression in happiness and achievement."

The Centennial meeting drew a large number of distinguished visitors from abroad, all bearing their organizations' congratulations to the AMA. Dr Fishbein served as master of ceremonies for many of the social and ceremonial functions at the centennial. Ironically, during what was one of the organization's happiest times, internal turmoil was building that would lead to his dismissal from the AMA staff 2 years later.

The end of the Fishbein era

While a clash of egos was probably a factor, the real issue in Fishbein's dismissal was his continued role as spokesperson for the AMA on virtually all issues, be they political or scientific. Some of the early national health insurance legislation — the Wagner-Murray-Dingell bill in 1943 and President Truman's 1945 proposals — had raised fears among some of the AMA's elected leadership that a more sophisticated response system as well as a much stronger Washington presence was needed. The AMA had opened its first Washington office in 1943, but it had little independence from Dr Fishbein and from the Chicago headquarters. As the 1940s progressed, Dr Fishbein survived at least two attempts to trim his sails, led in large part by the California delegation. These were efforts to confine Dr Fishbein's role to editing *JAMA,* eliminating him as the spokesman on political affairs. Truman's 1949 health legislation turned out to be the final straw, and Dr Fishbein rejected a final overture that would have permitted him to remain as editor. Therefore, the Board of Trustees presented the House of Delegates with a report announcing formal limits on the editor's activities and his upcoming retirement in December of that year. The action did not require House of Delegates action, but a reference committee called *JAMA* "an enduring monument" to Dr Fishbein's "genius and devotion."

Dr Fishbein opted to step down at once, creating a void in the AMA power structure that the organization struggled to define and fill for several years. Dr Fishbein himself would go on to lead an active professional life for many years, producing an auto-biography and serving for a time as editor of *Medical World News,* a weekly magazine that for several years competed actively with AMA publications. He died in 1976 at age 88.

In the Association's first 100 years, no decade had been as turbulent as the 1940s. The world, the nation, the practice of medicine, and the mood of the public all had undergone major changes. And the AMA had gone from an organization almost totally dedicated to science to one that was charging its members dues to allow funds for public relations, advertising, and lobbying. The perception of physicians, of the public, and of the media about the AMA had changed, and in the minds of some doctors, patients' attitudes toward them had hardened as well. The end of the decade might have marked the first time when physicians would begin looking wistfully back at the "good old days," but it was to be a dream that would not come true.

Exhibit sponsored by the AMA Council on Rural Health in the 1940s.

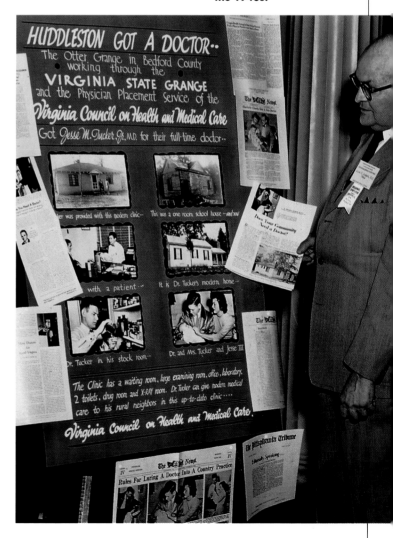

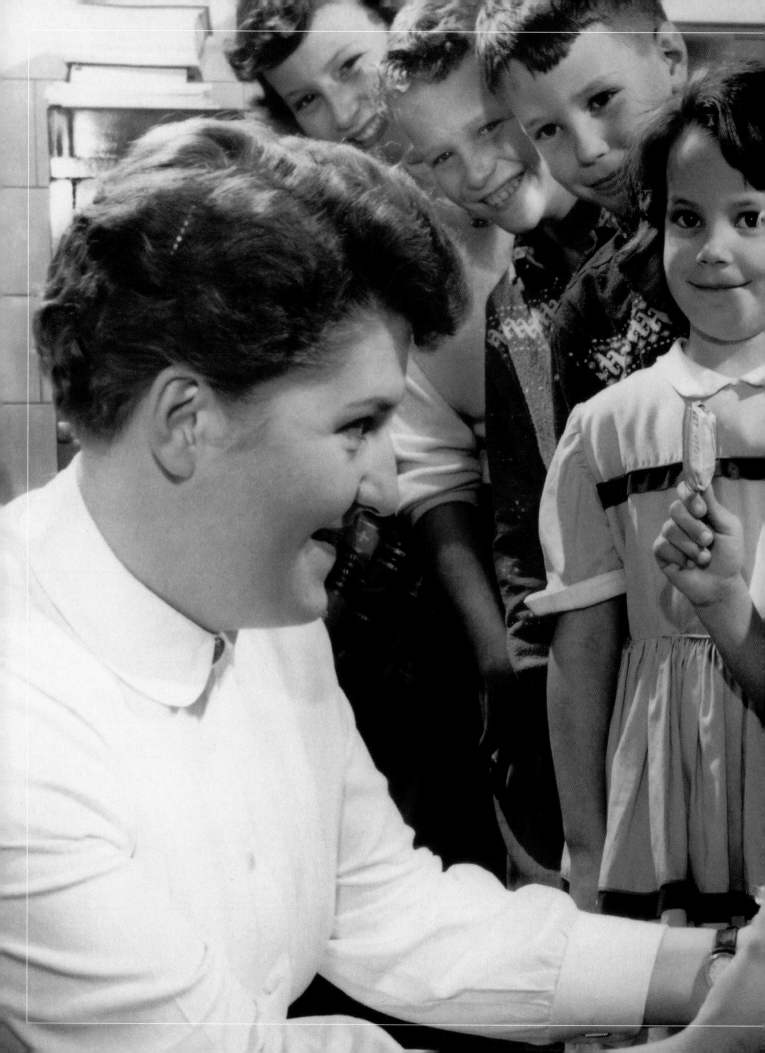

Chapter Six

The 1950s and 1960s

*A golden age for clinical medicine,
along with a political honeymoon
that ended in turmoil.*

6

The 1950s and 1960s

Dwight D. Eisenhower was President of the United States during much of the 1950s. His basically conservative administration, coupled with the generally conservative mood of the country, made the decade a quiet one for medicine — if the focus is solely on sweeping reform legislation. However, the decade began and ended in turmoil. At the same time, it was the beginning of a golden age for clinical medicine and patient care.

The 1950s began with the United States heavily involved in the Korean Conflict, which saw many physicians, including some who had served in World War II, on active duty in a far-off land. Despite the high casualty toll, the war — as had previous ones — led to major gains in medical care. Notably, the Korean Conflict was the first in which the helicopter played a major role. That machine was not developed with emergency medical care in mind, but the chopper's widespread use in Korea fostered the growth and success of the Mobile Army Surgical Hospital (M*A*S*H, as it became known to moviegoers and television watchers a generation later) and led to dramatic improvements in survival rates for battlefield casualties.

Overleaf: Polio vaccine eliminated one of the most feared diseases. This was a clinic in Milwaukee, Wis.

On the scientific front, the news was exciting. Consider these developments
in the early 1950s alone:

- **Jonas Salk, MD, administered his polio vaccine to 100 children. It
  was the beginning of the end for one of the most feared childhood
  diseases of the century.**

- **Isoniazid was discovered to be effective in treating tuberculosis.
  This would save thousands of lives and lead to the control of
  another of the nation's (and the world's) most feared diseases.**

- **On May 6, 1953, John H. Gibbon, Jr, MD, conducted the first
  successful use of a heart-lung machine, diverting the bloodstream
  of an 18-year-old patient while he repaired a heart defect. A
  year later, the first kidney transplant was performed.**

In a few years, the scope of medical practice would change dramatically.
The 1950s could well be considered the beginning of the "industrial
revolution" for medicine. The revolution was fueled by an explosion
of knowledge unprecedented at the time. It probably was not a mere
coincidence that this explosion was accompanied by the first uses of
computer technology to compile and analyze data, giving scientists yet
another powerful research tool (followed, in a few more years, by the
CT scanner and all its derivative devices).

Government's role in medical education and ethics

The growing emphasis on research led many medical schools to begin
transforming themselves into giant medical complexes. This created severe
town-and-gown controversies, as the traditional individual practitioners
battled what they saw as unfair competition from the government-aided
teaching institutions. The controversy was exacerbated by a major public
debate on the adequacy of the physician workforce at the time.

The AMA was resistant to expanding federal aid to medical schools, fearing
the accompanying imposition of federal regulations on curriculum and
academics. Some AMA foes termed this a smokescreen for a type of federal
birth control, and by 1951, the AMA House of Delegates endorsed a
matching grant program through which the federal government would
provide a one-time dose of bricks-and-mortar assistance to medical schools.
But concerns about medical schools and exactly where they fit into the
health care delivery system have continued to the present day.

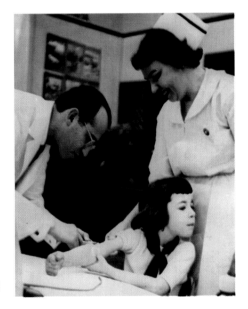

**Jonas Salk, MD,
administers the
polio vaccine he
developed to a
young patient.**

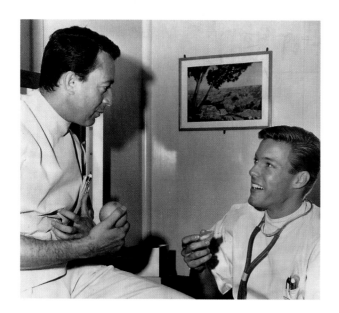

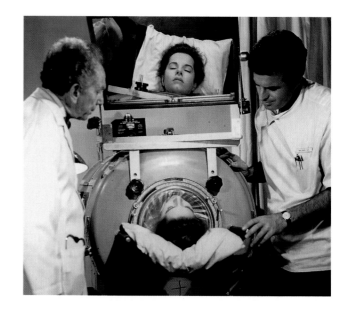

One manifestation in the 1950s was a controversy over "corporate practice," which had its roots in a 1912 AMA ethical statement that it was "unprofessional for a physician to dispose of his services under conditions that make it impossible to render adequate service to his patient." As this type of care became more widespread in the 1920s and 1930s, the AMA position strengthened. But in the 1950s, the issue became less clear-cut. What about patient care done in hospitals by salaried physicians? What

Changes in society's structure
brought a mini-revolution
to physicians' practice patterns.

about those salaried physicians in prepaid group insurance clinics? And what about care delivered in teaching hospitals by residents and salaried faculty members?

After several years of angry debate on the floor of the AMA House of Delegates, the issue was put to rest when the crucial passage of the Principles of Medical Ethics was amended to read: "…a physician should not dispose of his services under terms or conditions which tend to interfere with or impair the free and complete exercise of his medical judgment." This had

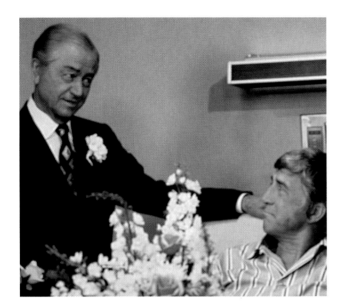

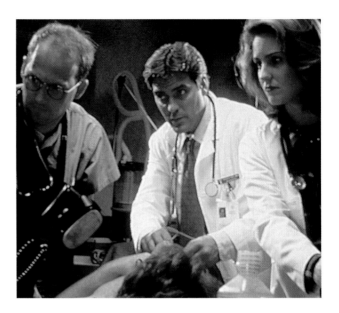

The public loved TV series about doctors. Above, from left, "Dr. Kildare," "Ben Casey," "Marcus Welby, MD," and a '90s descendant, "ER."

the effect of giving ethical sanction to any arrangement under which a physician had control over his/her medical decisions.

In 1959, the AMA went farther, adopting a report that addressed various forms of physician reimbursement. A key statement was the following:

> "The AMA believes that free choice of physician is the right of every individual and one which he should be free to exercise as he chooses. Each individual should be accorded the privilege to select and change his physician at will or to select his preferred system of medical care, and the AMA vigorously supports the right of the individual to choose between these alternatives."

Nearly 4 decades later, statements such as this one may seem elementary and not controversial, but in fact this was a milestone for organized medicine. However, it had little immediate impact on the animosities that many solo practitioners and not a few medical societies had developed toward institutional medicine.

The change in the ethical status of physicians practicing in institutions was just one feature of a complete revision of the Principles of Medical Ethics. This came after considerable wrangling on various ethical issues, including much discussion on the related topics of fee splitting, rebates, and commissions. At this point, the AMA's ethical code had evolved into a document of more than 5000 words that almost completely defied consistent interpretation. Therefore, at its 1957 meeting, the House of Delegates adopted a new 500-word set of Principles that was accompanied by a completely annotated series of opinions and reports of the Judicial

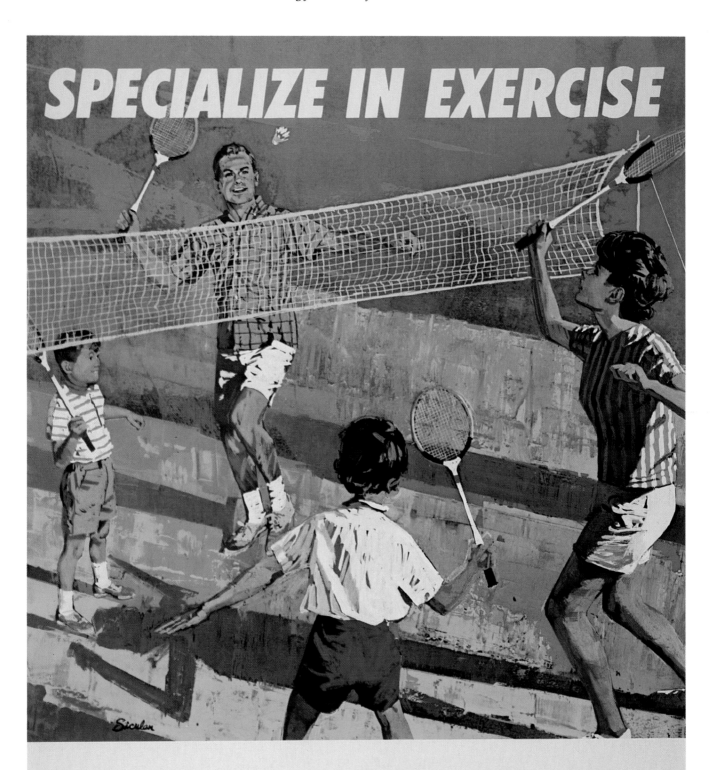

SPECIALIZE IN EXERCISE

For fun and fitness, make it a part of your family life.

You'll feel better • look better • sleep better.

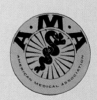

Council. This provided a new framework for the ethics of medicine, and, while the Principles were revised in 1980, the basic structure remains in place today.

Another major change in the 1950s was the acceptance of osteopathy, shunned by the AMA since osteopathy was recognized in 1874. However, as antibiotics began to come onto the scene in the 1930s, osteopathic schools began moving their teaching emphasis to more conventional medical science. After vigorous debate in the House of Delegates, the AMA stance was modified in 1959 to state that AMA members could ethically take part in the education of osteopathic physicians. This opened the door to MD-taught residency programs for graduates of schools of osteopathy and eliminated the AMA's long-time position that training in osteopathic schools lacked a scientific foundation.

The AMA strengthens its administration

Internally the AMA also was undergoing much turmoil. There was no strong central management. The committee and council structure was proliferating, and there was little administrative oversight. Activities in public relations and legislation were gaining momentum.

The AMA had responded to these changes and pressures in 1958 by replacing George F. Lull, MD, Dr Fishbein's successor, with F. J. L. (Bing) Blasingame, MD, as the organization's chief executive officer. The Texas physician, a former AMA Board of Trustees chair, undertook a major reorganization aimed at creating an effective management structure. His first step created a new organization along the lines of a more traditional corporation. He also greatly diminished the Board of Trustees' involvement in minute details of staff management, declaring that these were a proper function of staff managers.

Dr Blasingame also took on restructuring of the Washington office, putting in place strong individuals with a mandate to make direct contacts with key legislators. He presided over the birth of *The AMA News,* the predecessor to *American Medical News,* to explain to members what the AMA was doing, particularly in Washington. And he established a new field service division, headed by Aubrey D. Gates, a longtime friend of Arkansas Rep Wilbur Mills and a savvy politician in his own right.

All of this set the stage as the 1960s began and the Eisenhower years ended. In his last year in office, Eisenhower signed the Kerr-Mills law, supported by the AMA, which authorized federal grants to states to support state-run medical assistance programs for the needy elderly.

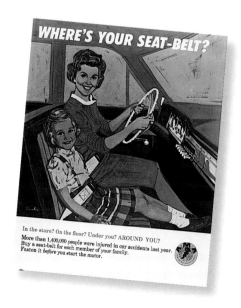

Public health education was an AMA priority in the 1950s, as the posters on these pages show.

This was the beginning of a turbulent period that brought John F. Kennedy and the New Frontier to the White House, the beginnings of the Vietnam War, the assassinations of Martin Luther King and Robert and John F. Kennedy, the swarm of protests and demonstrations that followed, and the election of Lyndon B. Johnson and the subsequent passage of Medicare and Medicaid. The first oral contraceptive, Enovid, was licensed in 1960 as well, opening the way to a new era of sexual freedom that, as events turned out, meshed perfectly with the mood of the country.

The creation of AMPAC and the fight against national health insurance

As the 1960s began, the AMA launched the American Medical Political Action Committee (AMPAC) to counteract the political efforts of the American Federation of Labor's Committee on Political Emphasis. Labor-backed national health legislation (the Forand bill) had failed in the late 1950s, but it was clear that with a Democratic administration assuming power, the stakes would rise. The formation of AMPAC led eventually to a fierce battle for power within the AMA that would have effects for 2 decades.

President Kennedy made an early, full-scale attempt at a national health insurance bill sponsored by Sen Clinton Anderson (D-NM) and Rep Cecil King (D-CA). Its target was Social Security retirees, who would have received 90 days of free hospital care and some nursing home care, but little in the way of physicians' services. The AMA's critical response was immediate and forthright, calling the legislation the "first major, irreversible step toward the complete socialization of medical care." The AMA statement, however, did not oppose aid to people in genuine need; it opposed compelling "one segment of our population to underwrite a socialized program of health care for another, regardless of need."

Edward R. Annis, MD, was AMA's most eloquent spokesperson in the 1960s battle over national health insurance.

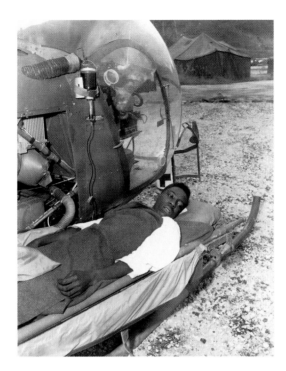

In a real-life scene that inspired a famous TV series, a US soldier wounded in Korea receives plasma en route by helicopter to a Mobile Army Surgical Hospital (MASH).

An all-out propaganda battle ensued, with both sides using advertising, public speeches, rallies, and a variety of grassroots activities. A high point of the White House campaign was a May 20, 1962, rally in Madison Square Garden, sponsored by the National Council on Senior Citizens for Health Care Through Social Security. President Kennedy was the featured speaker at the New York meeting; other rallies were scheduled in 20 other communities across the nation.

The AMA countered with one of its most celebrated responses, renting Madison Square Garden for use just after the Kennedy speech and filming a speech to the totally deserted arena by Edward R. Annis, MD, a dynamic Florida surgeon. The Annis speech was shown the next evening (the time was purchased by the AMA) on the NBC television network, and the result was a tremendous public relations coup for the AMA.

This may have been the turning point for the King-Anderson legislation. The crucial vote came on July 17 in the US Senate, which voted 52–48 to table a legislative amendment that would have brought the issue to a final vote in the Senate. This was a major setback for national insurance legislation.

The legislative battle began in earnest again in 1965, after Lyndon Johnson and the Democratic Congressional majority that swept into office on his coattails were in office. The King-Anderson proposal resurfaced. The AMA countered with Eldercare, a plan to provide comprehensive health benefits

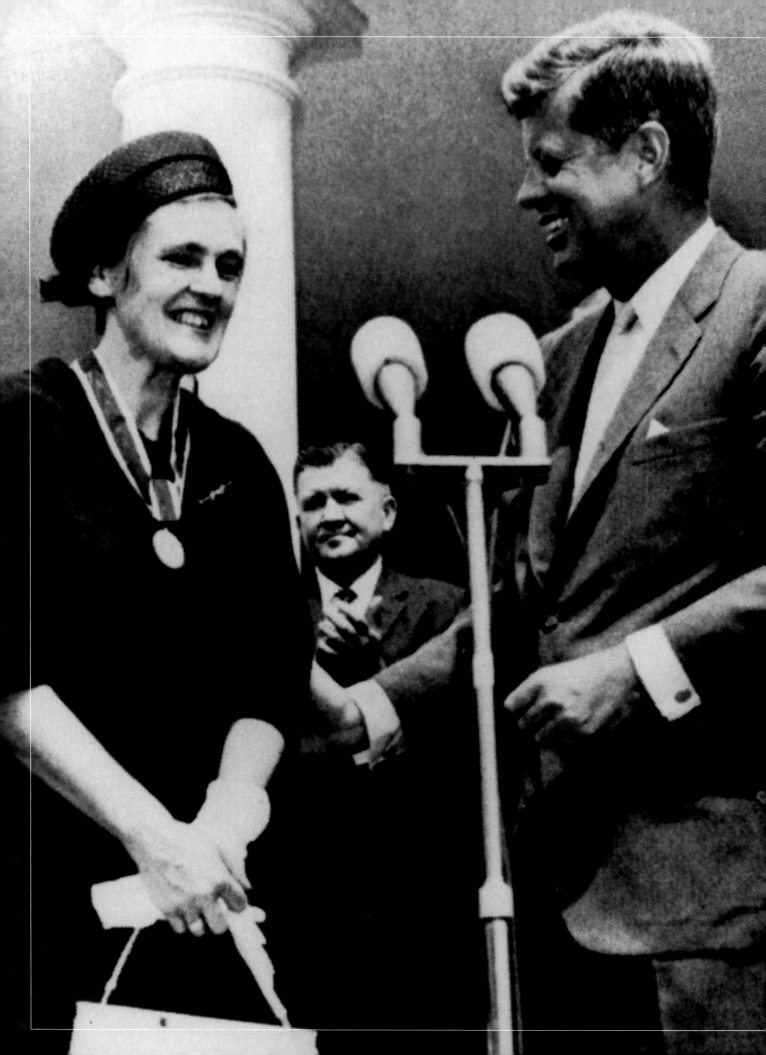

to the elderly needy. The situation was so critical that the AMA held a special House of Delegates meeting on February 6–7, 1965, to endorse formally the Eldercare proposal. While some delegates were voicing disapproval of the Board's legislative strategy, a new delegate from the Texas Medical Association, James H. Sammons, MD, rose and proposed a standing ovation for the Board for its handling of the situation. The resulting wave of applause silenced the critics, and Eldercare was endorsed.

However, Congressional hearings later that month produced a bill that contained three major features: Medicare Part A, based on the King-Anderson proposal; Medicare Part B, a supplementary, voluntary insurance plan covering physicians' services; and Medicaid, incorporating features of Eldercare and the Kerr-Mills law.

AMA's response to the new Medicare legislation

The AMA expressed opposition to the package. President Donovan Ward, MD, testified (with what turned out to be dead-on foresight) that "there is no totally effective method or methods which will keep the costs of the program under control."

However, votes were there to pass the legislation, and Ways and Means Committee Chairman Wilbur Mills of Arkansas, always sensitive to the political winds, pushed the measure through his committee. On April 8, 1965, the House passed the total bill. After final congressional action on July 28, President Johnson went to Independence, Mo, to sign the bill in the presence of former President Truman. At that point the AMA's leadership decided that the prudent course for patients and physicians would be to participate in the development of the regulations under which the new Medicare and Medicaid programs would function.

Anger over this turn of events led to another special session of the House of Delegates on October 2–3, 1965. There was angry talk of a boycott and more grumbling about the Board. The protesters' ardor was cooled somewhat by A. Leslie Hodson, an attorney retained by the AMA, who warned that while an individual physician could choose not to take part in Medicare, any formal group action would create severe antitrust problems. Then the AMA's new president, James Z. Appel, MD, of Pennsylvania, stated that a boycott would be "foolish and petulant," and added: "We are now expected by the public, the press, and the Congress to act as reasonable and mature men and women." (Dr Appel earlier had made similar comments during the AMA's June 1965 Annual Meeting in New York, a meeting that produced the legendary *New*

Facing page: The Food and Drug Administration's Frances Kelsey, MD, is honored by President John F. Kennedy in 1961 for her role in blocking approval of thalidomide, linked to birth defects.

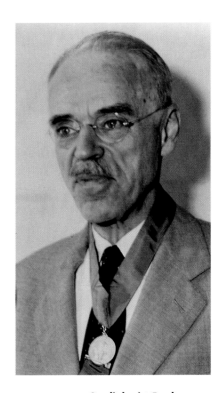

Cardiologist Paul Dudley White, President Dwight D. Eisenhower's physician, displays the AMA's Distinguished Service Award medal in 1952.

York Daily News headline reference to the "Biggest Doc Bash Ever." Coverage of Dr Appel's remarks in *The AMA News* brought a number of angry letters to the editor from physicians who opposed participation.)

The calm words of Dr Appel and others eventually carried the day, and the AMA took part in the development and implementation of Medicare. The AMA's predictions about escalating costs turned out to be true; at the same time, the dramatic increase in longevity in the United States also can be credited at least in part to Medicare.

Major issues of the 1960s, Medicare and the Vietnam War, *would have long-term impact.*

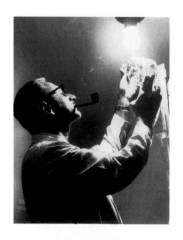

Albert Sabin, MD, developed the oral vaccine to prevent polio.

Medicare's passage had a long-term impact on the AMA and its leadership, as questions began to be raised about how to handle future legislative battles. The executive vice president, Dr Blasingame, was at ideological odds with some of the political activists involved in AMPAC. Dr Blasingame placed more emphasis on the scientific and scholarly role of the AMA; others sought more political action. The result was his ouster in 1968. The job went to his deputy for the previous 10 years, E. B. Howard, MD, touching off a major shift in direction for the organization.

Much of this was overlooked, for the public antipathy toward the war in Vietnam occupied center stage for the entire nation in the 1960s.

The unrest of the 1960s and AMA's response to the Vietnam War

At the AMA's meeting in San Francisco in June 1968, the Medical Committee for Human Rights seized the microphones at the opening session to shout their views at the delegates. A year later in New York, demonstrators again invaded the proceedings. One young physician burned what he said was his AMA membership card; House Speaker Russell Roth, MD, offered a cigarette lighter to assist him. (It turned out not to be an AMA membership card.) By 1970, however, the AMA had learned to deal more effectively with the protesters, offering them a special hearing room and an audience to which they could speak. The 1965 "Biggest Doc Bash" meeting also was the high-water mark for AMA scientific meetings. The growth of specialization would eventually see more and more physicians desert the AMA sessions for their own specialty organization's meeting. The AMA eventually halted these meetings in the 1970s.

On the international front, the AMA became involved in the Vietnam conflict through two major activities: the Volunteer Physicians for Vietnam program, in which physicians from this country served in Vietnamese communities treating both disease and war wounds suffered by innocent civilians, and a program to assist South Vietnam's medical schools. The AMA coordinated and administered this medical school project for nearly a decade, from 1966 to 1973.

In early 1970, Dr Howard, having been through 2 tumultuous years at the helm, gave a Boston audience his assessment of the AMA. He said the organization "has the resources, human and material, to promote the art and science of medicine and the betterment of the public health as its founders intended. Has it done so or has it failed? The answer is not an unqualified yes, for it has failed in some respects." One failure: not recognizing the escalating cost of care. Another: failure to anticipate the growing demand for care. His future goals for the AMA included aid to underserved areas, focusing attention on infant mortality problems, particularly among blacks, and moderating the AMA's conservative stand on abortion.

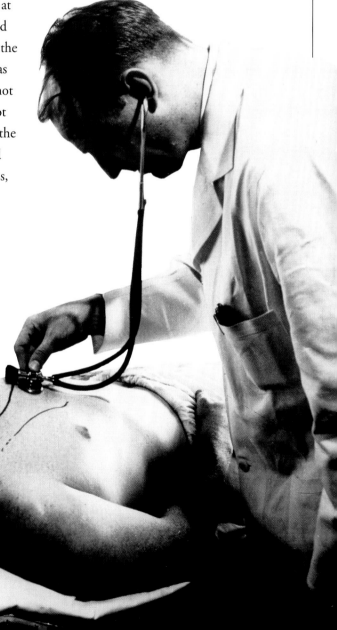

Luther Terry, MD, examines patient several years before he became US surgeon general and issued ground-breaking report on "Smoking and Health," 1964.

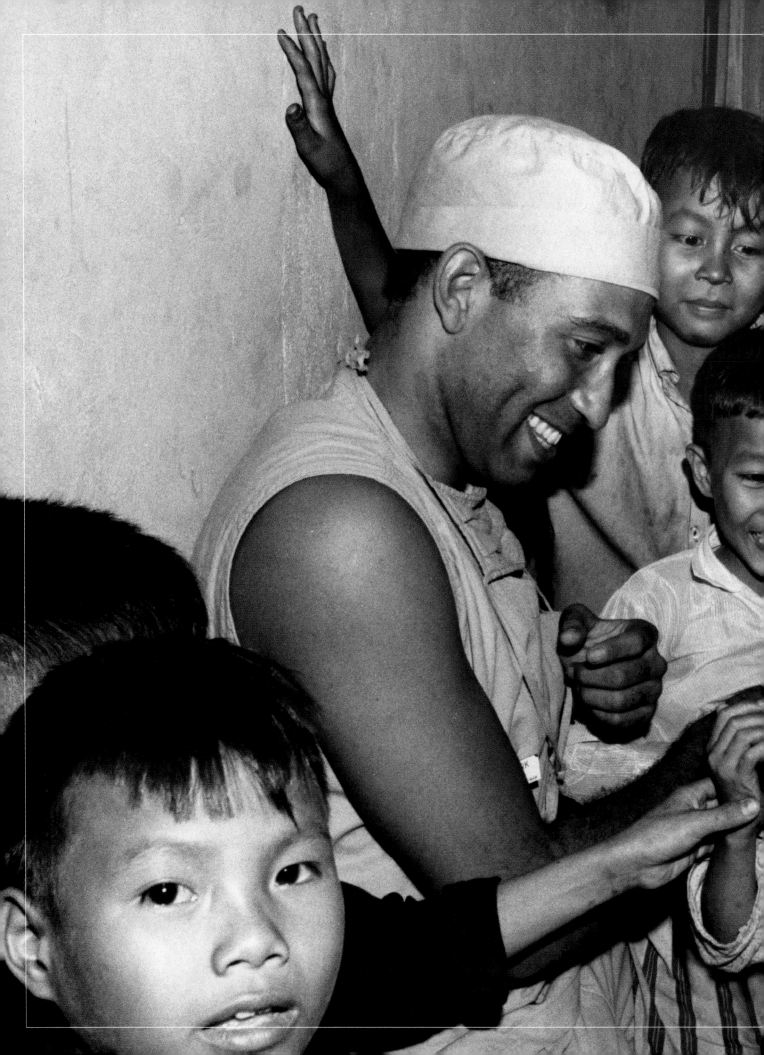

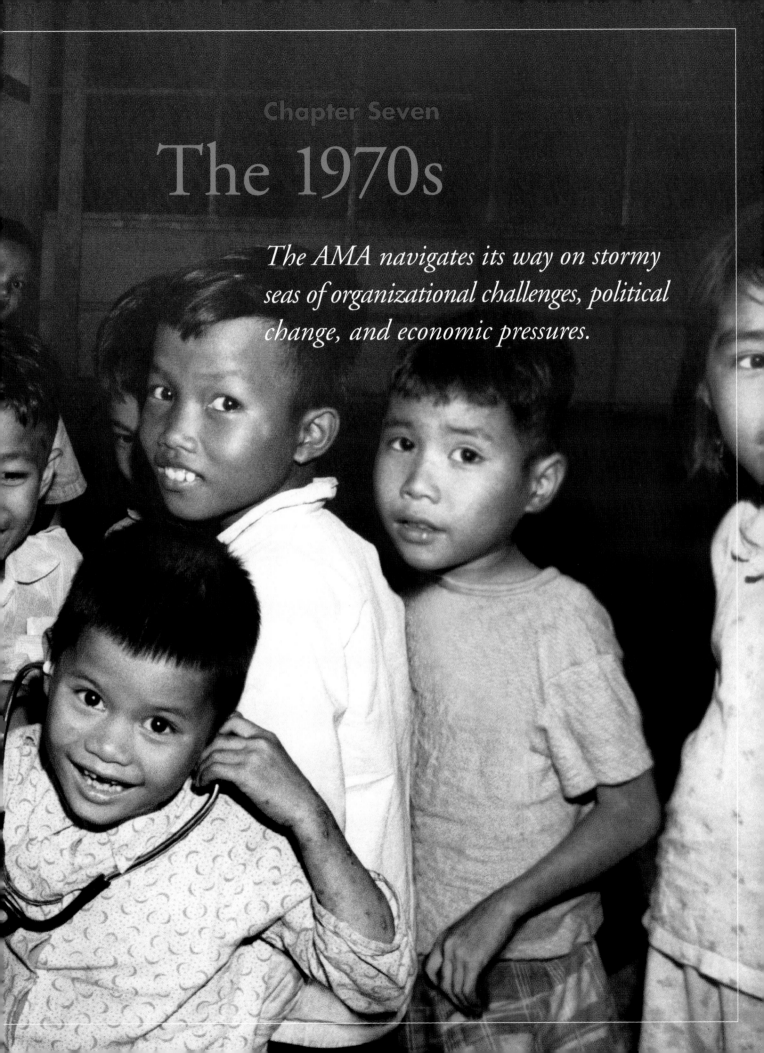

Chapter Seven

The 1970s

The AMA navigates its way on stormy seas of organizational challenges, political change, and economic pressures.

The 1970s

The turbulence that had marked much of the 1960s continued unabated in the early part of the 1970s. For the AMA, several factors converged to create organizational turmoil that eventually would change much of the structure of the organization.

The major problem was financial. The AMA House of Delegates, which sets the organization's membership dues each year, had been loath to increase dues. At the same time, the House had recognized the rapid changes in the way medicine was being practiced and the impact of government and outside influences, and was not reluctant to authorize and direct numerous new Association activities to respond.

During periods of prosperity for the AMA's publications, advertising revenues had supported many of the other activities of the organization. But this was not an area that offered unlimited growth. The House — reluctantly — had raised AMA dues in 1967 from $45 to $70. A year later the Board warned that inflation was adversely affecting the publishing operation. Beyond that, the Internal Revenue Service was taking aim at tax-exempt organizations' "unrelated business income," which included advertising revenues. By 1970, the AMA was operating at a deficit, and the Board proposed an $80 dues increase — to $150 a year — in 1971. The House balked and after some angry debate approved a $40 hike — not enough to eliminate the deficit. At the same

Overleaf: William Funderburk, MD, worked in Danang in 1967 as part of the AMA's Volunteer Physicians for Vietnam program.

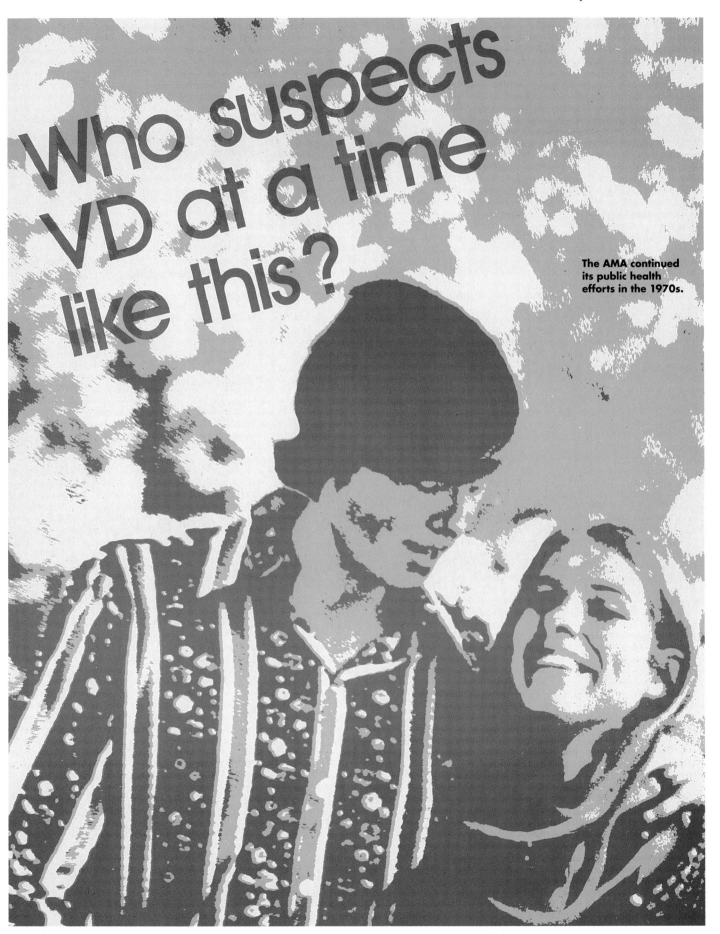

The AMA continued its public health efforts in the 1970s.

time, the House authorized an expensive public relations campaign. The result was a succession of deficit budgets; between 1970 and 1975, there was only 1 year (1972) of black ink.

Turbulent organizational politics and financial problems

Ernest B. Howard, MD, the executive vice president since 1968, reiterated his intent to retire in 1973 at age 65. This touched off a battle for the top staff job, with the decision ultimately coming down to a choice between Richard S. Wilbur, MD, and James H. Sammons, MD.

Dr Wilbur was the grandson of Ray Lyman Wilbur, MD, president of the AMA in 1923 and chair of the Council on Medical Education from 1929 to 1946; he was a nephew of Dwight L. Wilbur, MD, AMA president in 1968. The Wilbur family had impeccable Republican connections, particularly with Richard Nixon and Ronald Reagan. Dr Howard in 1969 had named Richard Wilbur as his top deputy, and Wilbur was granted a leave of absence from the AMA to serve in Washington as the US Assistant Secretary of Defense for Health and Environment. He was perceived by many as Dr Howard's heir apparent.

Medical practice in the '70s was moving in part to impersonal shopping-mall offices (opposite page), a marked change from the usual home office earlier in the century (right).

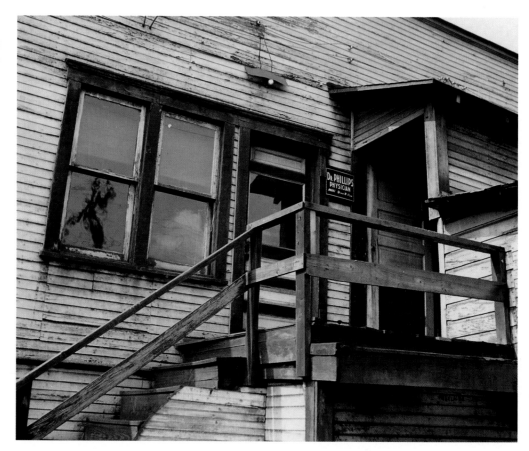

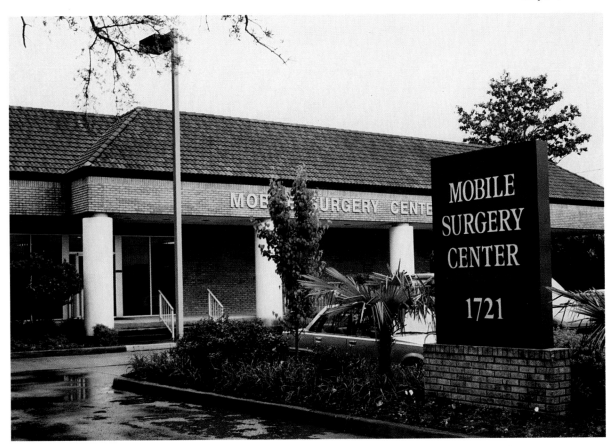

His primary challenger turned out to be Dr Sammons, the current Board chair and a man long active in AMA politics. A Baytown, Tex, family physician, he had been president of the Texas Medical Association and chair of the American Medical Political Action Committee's Board. He frequently would recall that he attended his first AMA meeting in 1948, while a medical student at St Louis University School of Medicine. "I saw people who were up on their feet and doing things. I thought it was a hell of an organization." On beginning practice, he immediately plunged into the activities of organized medicine, moving up rapidly from leadership positions at the county medical society level to the state and finally to AMA and AMPAC.

The Board in March of 1974 — on its 15th ballot — chose Dr Sammons as the new executive vice president. The action brought immediate charges from Dr Wilbur's supporters of political deal making. At the subsequent House of Delegates meeting, two incumbent members of the Board who reportedly had switched positions to support Dr Sammons were defeated. Dr Wilbur mounted a surprise candidacy for the position of AMA president-elect and wound up losing by only two votes to Max Parrott, MD, a former Board chair.

When the dust had settled, however, the political activities of those hectic 4 months left Dr Sammons firmly in charge, and he proceeded to make the most of the opportunity. His first task was to turn around the AMA's financial situation. The issue came to a head at the Interim Meeting in December 1974 in Portland, Ore. The Board had alerted the state delegations to the "critical financial situation" and had proposed a dues increase of $90, elimination of several councils and committees, cuts in the frequency of some of the publications, and other reductions in publishing costs. Staff cuts had dropped the number of AMA employees from 997 in August to 932 in December. This would produce a balanced budget of just over $35 million for 1975.

The Portland meeting of the House of Delegates was a donnybrook. A Reference Committee chaired by Joseph T. Painter, MD, coolly spent a long day listening to delegates express dismay over many of the proposals — particularly the dues increase — and voice misgivings over the board's handling of the situation. Eventually, the delegates approved a one-time $60 assessment to stabilize the Association's finances, then restored the old council structure on an interim basis while a special committee of the House studied the situation for 6 months.

This AMA exhibit helped train police in testing suspected drunken drivers.

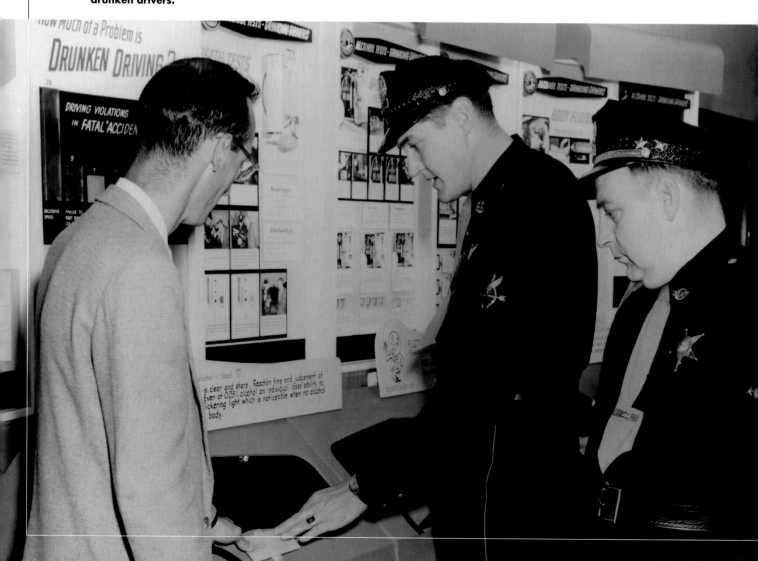

This special committee was headed by Dr Painter, a Texas internist who would go on to become AMA president and Board chair. The committee spent the time before the June 1975 meeting poring over AMA records, documents, and financial statements, and produced a detailed report that laid the framework for the organization for the next decade.

By the time of the meeting, almost 120,000 of the AMA's 170,000 members had paid the $60 assessment, easing the financial pinch. Nevertheless, there had been drastic curtailments in operations and major staff reductions of employees to 824.

With this background, Dr Painter and his committee went before the House with a detailed report. Its findings basically affirmed the Board's analysis of the problem — the analysis that the House had refused to accept in Portland. The report called for a substantial (but unspecified) dues increase, the discontinuance of *Prism* (a 2-year-old socioeconomic magazine), and major revisions in the council-committee structure. The House agreed with much of the Committee's report and enthusiastically adopted a dues increase to $250. At the same time, the first serious recognition was given to the need for ongoing, effective membership recruitment and retention programs. Perhaps most importantly, the House adopted the recommendation that basically disbanded two councils and 18 committees of the Board as well as 10 committees that reported to existing Councils.

Years later, Dr Sammons would look back and see long-term benefits from the financial crisis of 1974–1975, because the financial problems permitted the elimination of what he referred to as "fiefdoms." Without financial pressures, he said, "The change in direction, in management, [and] in the way policy is developed [was] a landmark in the history of the AMA. Retrospectively, the financial crisis, in my view, turned out to be the best thing that happened to the AMA in 50 years."

American Medical News headlines reflected major issues of the '70s.

New members and new social issues

Financial affairs were not the only issues in the 1970s, however. In a major step toward attracting younger members, the House of Delegates had opened AMA membership to medical students and residents in 1972. In that same year, the AMA fired the opening salvo in what would become an all-out war on smoking and tobacco products, urging the federal government to reduce and control the use of tobacco products and supporting legislation that would prohibit dispensing of samples of tobacco products.

A year later would come the US Supreme Court's landmark *Roe v Wade* decision legalizing abortion. At the Annual Meeting that June, the House of Delegates approved the following statement that remains as AMA policy today:

1. **Abortion is a medical procedure and should be performed only by a duly licensed physician and surgeon in conformance with standards of good medical practice and the Medical Practice Act of his state.**

2. **No physician or other professional personnel shall be required to perform an act violative of good medical judgment. Neither physician, hospital, nor hospital personnel shall be required to perform any act violative of personally held moral principles. In these circumstances, good medical practice requires only that the physician or other professional withdraw from the case, so long as the withdrawal is consistent with good medical practice.**

Looking ahead to 1991, the House approved the following statement regarding abortion that emphasizes the traditional physician-patient relationship:

It is the policy of the AMA to strongly condemn any interference by the government or other third parties that causes a physician to compromise his or her medical judgement as to what information or treatment is in the best interest of the patient.

The science of medicine continued to march forward dramatically during the 1970s. New drugs were making inroads on hypertension, on various mental disorders, on ulcers, and on many cardiac conditions. Improved technology, including computed tomography (CT scanning), was making possible surgery undreamed of only a few years earlier. In 1975, the American College of Surgeons and the American Surgical Association collaborated on the *Study on Surgical Services for the United States,* which attempted to evaluate on the basis of cost-effectiveness some of the advances in surgical technique. It analyzed 64 leading contributions to surgical research between 1945 and 1970. It concluded that through the development of just 15 of those procedures, some 78,000 lives had been saved in 1970 alone, and that the resultant savings in costs were some 60 times the cost of the research.

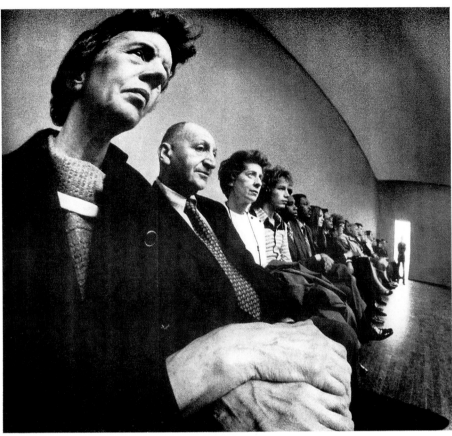

The day everybody had to see a doctor.

We have nightmares about it.

That awful, impossible day. When the routine aches, the vague ills, the serious injuries, the disasters all come together. When everybody in America might suddenly need a doctor. And there aren't enough doctors to go around.

It isn't pleasant to think about. But we're doctors. It's our job to think about the unthinkable.

Because the fact is, there's a shortage of doctors now. America has only 278,000 physicians taking care of patients. One of us for 818 of you.

Because *we're* outnumbered, *you* could lose.

The story used to be that doctors deliberately kept their own numbers down. To keep their fees up.

But the doctor shortage is hurting doctors as much as anybody.

It's stretching the capacity of our profession dangerously thin.

One cure is more doctors. And we are working on it. In the last nine years, $48 million worth of medical student loans have been guaranteed by America's doctors (through their professional organization, the American Medical Association).

And today, over 7,500 students are in medical school or intern/residency programs with the help of loans guaranteed by the A.M.A.—Education and Research Foundation.

What of the medical schools themselves? America's doctors have given them $50 million just since 1962.

We're making progress. While the overall population has grown 12% since 1960, the physician population has grown 28%.

You see, there are going to be a lot more of you in the future.

And we want to be sure there are a lot more of us to take care of you.

America's Doctors of Medicine

This AMA public service advertisement warned of the need for more physicians.

The reemergence of national health legislative battles

The 1970s also saw a sustained effort by Sen Edward Kennedy (D-Mass) to achieve national health insurance. He began in August of 1970, charging that there was a "crisis in the availability and delivery of essential health service" and arguing that the United States was "the only industrial nation that does not have a national health service or a program of national health insurance." The AMA countered with its own legislation, called Medicredit.

Dr Parrott, then the Board chair, took on Kennedy's charges at a 1971 hearing of the Senator's health subcommittee, stating: "…you might consider the US record on infant mortality. In 1940 there were 47 deaths per thousand live births; in 1950, 29.2; in 1960, 26; and in June 1971, 19.2. That is better than a 25 percent drop just in the last decade." Further, life expectancy at birth had risen from 62.9 years in 1940 to 70.8 years in 1970. "We *are* making progress," Dr Parrott said.

Eventually, the 1970s ended with no national health legislation ever emerging from a Congressional committee. The legislative spotlight was monopolized instead by the enactment of legislation in 1972 that created Professional Standards Review Organizations (PSROs). The legislation borrowed some principles of peer review but its target was cost surveillance, and the medical profession wanted no part of it. However, the AMA was in somewhat the same political position as it had been when Medicare was enacted; open disobedience of the law of the land was not politically realistic.

Robert B. Hunter, MD, later to be an AMA Board chair and president, was given the somewhat thankless job of heading an advisory committee to work with the US Department of Health, Education, and Welfare to implement the program. Grassroots efforts favoring repeal of the entire piece of legislation gathered steam, however, and reached a climax at the House of Delegates meeting in December 1973 in Anaheim, Calif. A stormy debate and complex political maneuverings would result in adoption of a milder resolution calling for the AMA to seek constructive amendments to the legislation. Jousting over the program and its impact continued for nearly a decade, and in 1980 the AMA House finally voted to seek repeal. The next year, in the absence of any proof that significant economies were being achieved, Congress started to phase out the program.

This battle was going on at the same time that the Nixon administration was launching the Health Maintenance Act, which it billed as a way to encourage market competition rather than imposing regulations on medical care costs. Congress in 1973 authorized spending $375 million over a 5-year period to develop HMOs. In 1974, Congress put into place a complicated, bureaucratic planning process by creating 204 Health Systems Agencies. This was an effort doomed to failure, and Congress put it to death in the early 1980s.

AMA worked to influence debate on **peer review, cost control, availability of care** *in Congress in the 1970s.*

AMA helps in the search for solutions to the rising cost of medical care

The nation's concern with rising expenditures for medical care could not be ignored, and the AMA moved to take the lead in the search for solutions. The AMA organized the National Commission on the Cost of Medical Care in 1975 and charged it with developing ideas to stabilize health care costs. The panel, chaired by former AMA President Max Parrott, MD, was impressive, with representatives of business, labor, government, and academia joining physician leaders. The commission was independent of the AMA and given the latitude to develop its own proposed solutions.

What emerged was a series of 48 recommendations covering a broad scope of issues. The first eight, however, addressed cost consciousness among consumers and providers and, in the context of the times, were considered revolutionary by many physicians. These included calls for consumer cost sharing; more tightly run health insurance programs; HMOs and fair market competition among competing delivery systems; informational directories of providers; and experiments with new methods of financing care through the use of hospital or physician groups that could demonstrate an ability to deliver quality care at below-average cost. Two key passages from the report:

> *"Some mechanisms must be put in place to assure that no group of consumers is denied quality care due to inability to pay."*

> *"The commission believes that the greatest hope for cost containment in the provision of health care lies in strengthening price consciousness in the health care marketplace."*

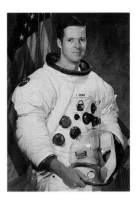

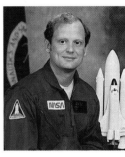

MD-astronaut Joseph Kerwin (top) in the 1970s paved the way for other MD-astronauts such as Norman Thagard, MD (bottom), in the 1990s.

Meanwhile, Jimmy Carter was elected president, and his administration in 1977 proposed capping hospital charges. Congress — perhaps recalling the failure of President Nixon's wage/price control effort in 1971 — wouldn't go along. However, Carter's proposal did motivate the AMA to join with major hospital organizations to create the Voluntary Effort, which, as the name implies, sought voluntary solutions to health care inflation.

As the decade ended, the pressures to control costs seemed to beset the medical profession from all sides. There were new clinical challenges ahead as well. At a time when many of the once-feared communicable diseases had been eliminated, a new epidemic was just around the corner — one that has eluded a cure or vaccine for 15 years. While the scientific search is frustrating, the AIDS epidemic has served again to illuminate the AMA's role in communicating information to the public and to the profession.

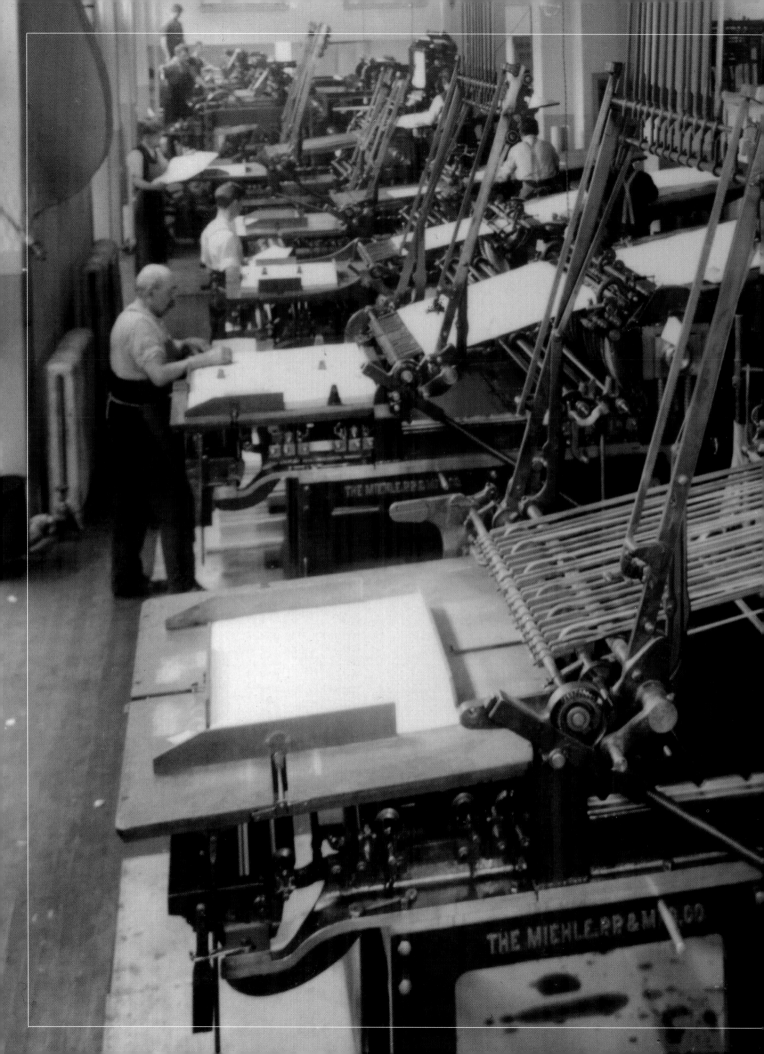

Chapter Eight

Publishing

The AMA began its publishing activities with JAMA in the 1800s. Today, it is the largest medical publisher in the world.

Publishing

8

For more than a century, the AMA has published the *Journal of the American Medical Association.* This venerable publication has served the Association well in many areas: as a method of communicating with physicians, as a communications tool to the media and thus to the public at large, as a membership benefit, and as a major source of revenue. The founding of *JAMA* marked the beginning of the AMA's entry into the publishing world; today, the Association produces not only *JAMA* but also nine specialty journals and the influential socioeconomic weekly newspaper, *American Medical News.* Consumer books as well as various technical and educational publications for physicians are also a major part of the AMA's publishing activity. In addition to their role as a source of information for patients and the profession, AMA's publications are a significant source of Association revenue. In 1996, the AMA received some $95 million from its sale of advertising, subscription fees, and sales of other books and products. Equally important, through its publishing activities the AMA communicates with its members and with millions of patients and physicians all over the world.

The founding of *JAMA* stemmed in large measure from the inspiration of Lewis A. Sayre, MD, the AMA's president in 1880. He was not impressed by the AMA's annual publication of the transactions of its meeting and was frankly envious of the success of the *British Medical Journal,* published by

Overleaf: For many years, the AMA operated its own printing plant. This view shows the equipment used about 1905.

the British Medical Association. His enthusiasm for change set in motion the chain of events that led to publication of the first issue of *JAMA* on July 14, 1883. The editor was Nathan S. Davis, MD — the same Dr Davis who had been the AMA's principal founder nearly 40 years earlier.

Dr Davis and a series of other physicians led *JAMA* through its initial growing pains, but the appointment in 1899 of George H. Simmons, MD, as editor truly put the publication on the road to greatness. In 1901, at the time of the major reorganization of the AMA, he became its secretary and later its general manager.

During his tenure as editor, Dr Simmons was unsparing and unrelenting in his attacks on the advertising of fraudulent remedies and patent medicines and played a major part in the campaign against proprietary medical schools. These activities incurred a great deal of wrath among the targets of the campaigns, but he and *JAMA* were undeterred. In his *History of the American Medical Association 1847 to 1947,* Dr Fishbein was unstinting in his praise of Dr Simmons, lauding "the tremendous part that he played in the reorganization of the American Medical Association in 1901, in the establishment of its *Journal* and headquarters office on a superlative business basis and in creating a firm foundation on which his successors were able to erect the tremendous and efficient organization that exists today."

One noteworthy innovation under Dr Simmons' guidance was the first publication of licensure examination results on a state-by-state basis — a milestone in raising educational standards. He also took the lead in organizing the Council on Medical Education and Hospitals and in launching the Department of Propaganda for Reform (later the Bureau of Investigation), which was the AMA's vehicle for the attack on fraud and quackery. Dr Simmons took part in the organization of the AMA Council on Pharmacy and Chemistry, which he later chaired. He also began publication of the *American Medical Directory,* now in its 31st edition.

Morris Fishbein's strong leadership aided the growth of *JAMA*

His successor, Morris Fishbein, MD, had the advantage of working for Dr Simmons for 11 years after joining the *JAMA* staff in 1913, fresh out of Chicago's Rush Medical College. In 1924 he was named to succeed Dr Simmons, beginning a reign of 25 years during which he achieved power and public stature probably unmatched by any physician in this century. Not only the editor but also the organization's general secretary, he was medicine's public spokesman on everything from science to quackery

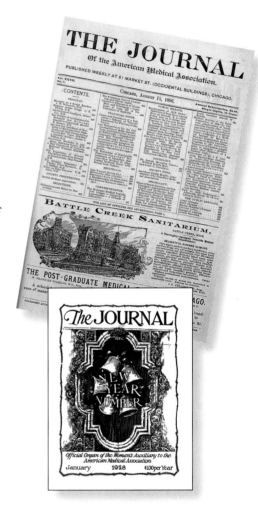

Early editions of **JAMA** featured advertising on the cover page (top). By 1928, the AMA's Woman's Auxiliary had its own journal.

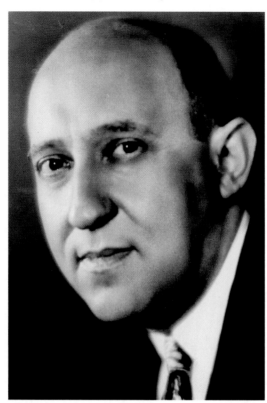

Famed JAMA editor Morris Fishbein, MD, was instrumental in building the publication's quality and reputation.

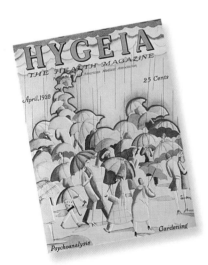

This 1928 *Hygeia* cover was designed to catch the eye of consumers.

to politics. A 1947 *Time* cover story called him — in that magazine's inimitable style — "the nation's most ubiquitous, the most widely maligned, and perhaps most influential medico."

In addition to *JAMA,* he presided over nine monthly specialty journals (diseases of children, dermatology, general psychiatry, internal medicine, neurology, ophthalmology, otolaryngology, surgery, and pathology). He also was responsible for the rapid growth of *Hygeia,* which was founded in 1923 and later became *Today's Health.* This monthly magazine was devoted to the health education of the public with the side effect of serving as a public relations tool. *Reader's Digest* and other national magazines frequently reprinted its articles, and newspapers culled its pages for quotable material. In the 1970s, there was even a half-hour "Today's Health" TV show.

Financial woes eventually killed *Today's Health,* however. It was a benefit of AMA membership, meaning there was an extensive circulation without direct reimbursement. Its high advertising standards made it vulnerable to the growing number of consumer and women's magazines that sprang up after

Facing page: This *Hygeia* cover from 1926 promotes the advantages of exercise and fitness. *Hygeia* later became *Today's Health.*

HYGEIA

A JOURNAL OF INDIVIDUAL AND COMMUNITY HEALTH

Published by the American Medical Association

535 N. Dearborn St., Chicago

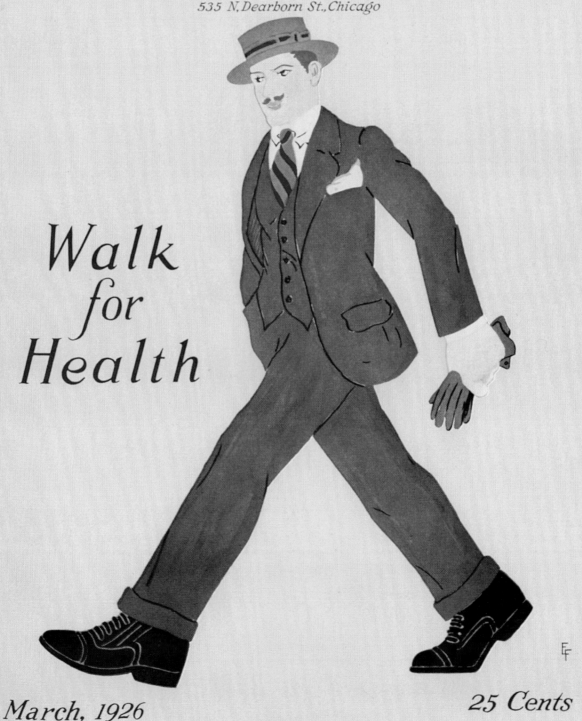

Walk for Health

March, 1926

25 Cents

JAMA

THE JOURNAL of the American Medical Association

March 7, 1977

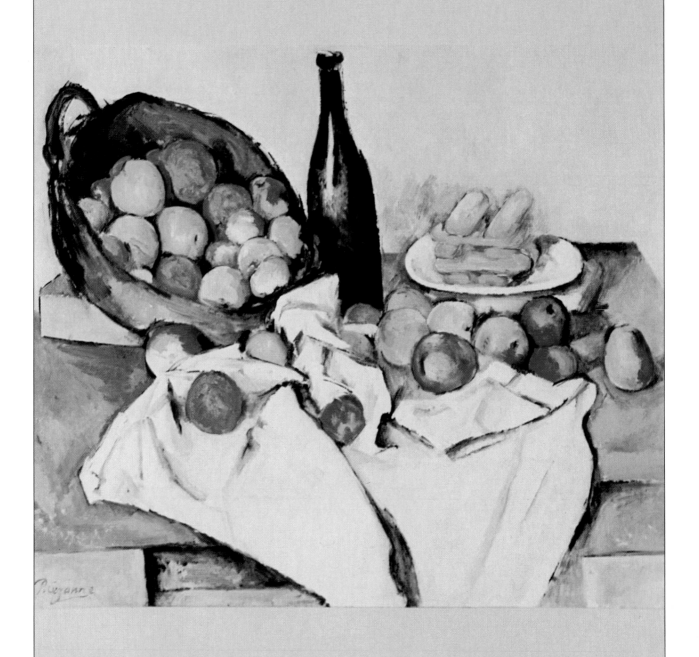

World War II, and in 1976 — during the AMA's bleakest financial period — the Board of Trustees sold the magazine to Family Communications, Inc, which published *Family Health.* The AMA was paid $200,000, and Family Communications assumed liability for $1.4 million worth of prepaid, unfulfilled circulation.

At the time of Dr Fishbein's ouster from the AMA in 1949, *JAMA* was riding high. There was little competition for advertisers or readers. Subscription and advertising revenues from AMA's publications in 1949 totaled $2.4 million, which would finance a year's activities for the entire AMA, making membership dues more or less superfluous. This success was not a fluke. Dr Fishbein's editorship created a lively, witty, aggressive publication that ranged across science, medicine, and research — with a regular dose of humor thrown in. There was also the AMA "Seal of Acceptance," a Fishbein innovation based on the AMA's own evaluation of products through its Councils on Pharmacy and Chemistry, Physical Therapy, and Foods and Nutrition — a powerful incentive to advertisers.

Dr Fishbein himself was a trenchant commentator. A typical example of his writing attacked the report of the prestigious Committee on the Costs of Medical Care in the 1930s, seeing: "…on one side the forces representing the great foundations, public health officialdom, social theory — even socialism and communism — inciting to revolution; on the other side, the organized medical profession…urging an orderly evolution." Another sentence began, "The rendering of all medical care by groups or guilds or medical soviets…."

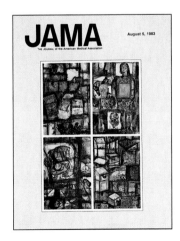 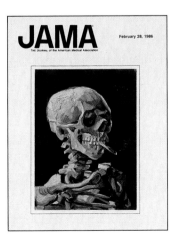 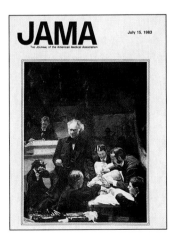

Since 1964, *JAMA's* covers have carried reproductions of artwork linked to current medical issues by famous artists such as Paul Cezanne (facing page) and (from left) Ire and Toshi Maruki, Vincent Van Gogh, and Thomas Eakins.

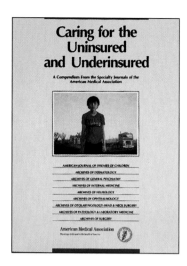 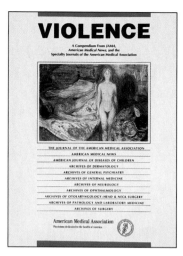

Compendiums of material from AMA publications have focused on specific problems of society such as indigent care and domestic violence.

New strategies and directions

It was, in fact, Dr Fishbein's political stridency that helped lead to his demise at the AMA. His successor, Austin Smith, MD, inherited a successful publication, however, and chose to steer a different course. The AMA itself was changing — the fellowship concept gave way to membership dues with *JAMA* as a benefit of membership — and the AMA was becoming increasingly involved in political action. Dr Smith, the former staff secretary of the Council on Pharmacy and Chemistry, lacked his predecessor's flair. He also shifted *JAMA*'s focus somewhat away from science and research and toward more coverage of organizational activities, including numerous (and occasionally voluminous) reports prepared by AMA councils and committees.

In 1959 the Board of Trustees appointed as editor John H. Talbott, MD, an experienced medical editor and a professor of medicine at the University of Buffalo. He did not wait long to make major changes. One symbolic move was to eliminate advertising from the front cover, calling this "the initial presentation to the medical profession of the philosophy of the current regime for improvement of the scientific publications of the AMA." He began the use of four-color reproductions of works of art on the *JAMA* cover in 1964 — a practice that has continued since that time.

Dr Talbott's successes and innovations, however, came at a time when market conditions for all publications were unfavorable, and revenues sank from $13.6 million in 1967 to $11.9 million in 1968 and $10 million in 1969, the year in which Dr Talbott stepped down to become editor emeritus. His successor, Hugh H. Hussey, MD, had been dean of Georgetown Medical School and chair of the AMA Board. A thoughtful, precise, and scholarly man, Dr Hussey continued generally on the course set by Dr Talbott, including severe restrictions of material from AMA councils.

Dr Hussey's retirement for health reasons in 1973 brought to the editorship Robert Moser, MD, who arrived with an agenda that included the launching of international editions and increased emphasis on continuing education activities. He created an advisory board to help with outreach to major scientific institutions, improving the quality of manuscripts being submitted. He also launched *JAMA en Español* with a Spanish publisher and eyed expansion of that edition into Latin America. However, he resigned rather than accede to the 1975 budget reductions. His successor, William Barclay, MD, had headed the AMA Division of Scientific Activities for 5 years and previously had been a professor of medicine at the University of Chicago. Dr Barclay was familiar with the AMA's internal structure and with the world of clinical practice. In his 7-year tenure, he targeted *JAMA* to the practicing physician, staying "in the forefront of medical science in those areas that could be understood by the majority of physicians," he said later.

JAMA expands to reach international readers

Dr Barclay also played a major role in the overseas expansion of the publication. Starting in 1976, five Spanish-language editions of *JAMA* were developed for Mexico, Central America, Colombia, Venezuela, and Argentina. Steps were being taken for further expansion in South America, but the sagging international economy drove the AMA's Spanish publisher into bankruptcy.

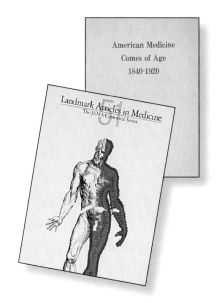

Marking its centennial, JAMA published a compendium (above) of landmark articles. Meanwhile, longtime staff editor Lester King, MD, authored a major history (top).

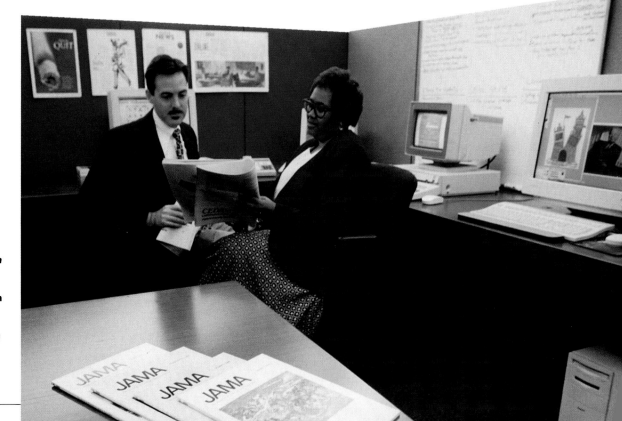

JAMA and American Medical News are weeklies with a combined circulation of some 625,000, both produced in a high-tech publishing operation at AMA headquarters.

The international expansion of *JAMA,* however, was just beginning to gather momentum. In the late 1970s, the AMA made a corporate decision to expand the international role of *JAMA.* Working through royalty arrangements with foreign medical publishers, the AMA began publishing editions of *JAMA*

Reassuming an earlier role, JAMA *has become a trenchant commentator* on social issues and public health issues.

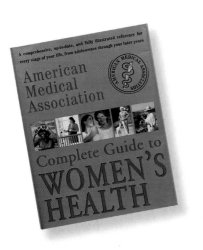

The AMA Complete Guide to Women's Health was published in 1996.

in French, German, Flemish, and Japanese, with monthly distribution in much of Europe and in Japan. The AMA also collaborated with the Chinese Medical Association in Beijing to produce a bimonthly Chinese-language edition of *JAMA* in the People's Republic of China. By 1996, there would be 21 international editions of *JAMA* and 18 international editions of the specialty journals.

The early 1980s also saw the retirement of Dr Barclay, who had done much to upgrade the AMA's scientific publications, and the arrival on the scene of *JAMA*'s 14th editor, George D. Lundberg, MD. Dr Lundberg moved immediately to put his stamp on the publication. He expanded the role of peer reviewers but also insisted that the publication should be enjoyable as well as educational. A mission statement published early in his career summed up his philosophy: "We feel that a physician, if he reads only *JAMA* for a year but reads every issue cover to cover, should not, at the end of the year, be out of touch with anything in the general medical field. That is what we try to do."

Under Dr Lundberg, *JAMA* has reassumed its role as an aggressive commentator on social and political issues. *JAMA* articles in recent years have evaluated various proposals for health system reform, graded the nation's progress (or lack thereof) in combating violence, and extensively attacked the tobacco industry. *JAMA* remains a major source of information for the nation's news media as well. This is in large part the result of an aggressive communications campaign that distributes a press packet covering each issue of *JAMA* to 2500 science and health reporters around the world via mail, facsimile, or e-mail. A weekly video news release on *JAMA*'s lead story is available by satellite to every TV station in the United States.

Reporting on news of the profession

The vigorous growth of *JAMA* in the 1980s was paralleled by a strong performance by *American Medical News,* the AMA's weekly newspaper. Founded in 1958 as a twice-a-month tabloid called *The AMA News,* with the principal goal of informing physicians about the AMA's position on national health insurance, the publication initially devoted itself to reporting on organizational matters and to strong criticism of pending national health legislation. The *News* became a weekly in 1965, and in 1969 — as part of an overall revamping of AMA's communications structure — the paper became *American Medical News,* with the specific mandate to report news of general interest to the profession, rather than serving primarily as a "house organ." The real growth of the *News* actually began in 1971 with the decision to accept pharmaceutical advertising; initially this publication featured consumer-product ads for automobiles, office equipment, travel, etc.

American Medical News struggled through the AMA's economic problems of the 1970s along with the rest of the Association. As the decade ended, however, the *News* became one of the first medical publications to offer its advertisers the opportunity to publish demographic packages that allowed them to target their products to physicians in certain specialties or groups of specialties. This capability put the newspaper into a much more favorable competitive position with for-profit publications targeted to specific specialties, and with its two major competitors for the nonclinical audience, *Medical Economics* and *Medical World News.* In addition to a jump in advertising revenue, *American Medical News'* growth enabled the editors to expand

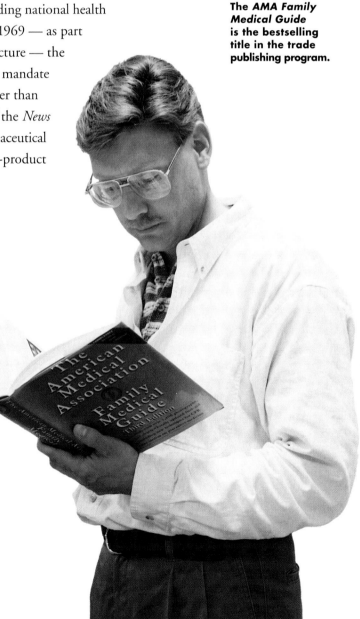

The *AMA Family Medical Guide* is the bestselling title in the trade publishing program.

Washington coverage and to launch new regular sections devoted to the business aspects of the health care industry (once the sole purview of *Medical Economics*) and of the personal, human side of medical practice.

AMA works with major publishers to provide clear, accurate health information to consumers.

A comprehensive consumer publication program

Also in the 1980s, the AMA reentered the world of consumer publishing. After the sale of *Today's Health* (the successor to *Hygeia*) in 1976, the AMA had targeted new approaches to reaching patients. In the early 1980s, the AMA and Random House published a set of "Straight-Talk, No-Nonsense Guides" on the subjects of sleep, back care, women's health, and the health of people over age 50. The major step was taken in 1982, when the AMA and Random House published the first edition of the *AMA Family Medical Guide,* which has been one of the organization's most successful ventures (and which was published on CD-ROM in 1995).

Overall the AMA has sold some 15 million consumer books on topics ranging from first aid to women's health to sleep. Recent titles have included the *AMA Encyclopedia of Medicine,* a comprehensive reference book; *AMA Handbook of First Aid and Emergency Care,* revised in 1990 as a comprehensive, step-by-step illustrated guide to dealing with injuries, illnesses, and medical emergencies; the *AMA Home Medical Library,* a lavishly illustrated 19-volume series marketed exclusively through direct mail by the Reader's Digest that covered a variety of health topics; a series of books for children aged 3 to 7; the *AMA Guide to Prescription and Over-the-Counter Drugs,* published in 1989 and covering more than 4000 drugs; a set of pocket guides to emergency first aid, sports first aid, back pain, and calcium, published in 1994–1995 with Random House; the *AMA Guide to Your Family's Symptoms,* containing a series of self-help charts; and *Seven Weeks to Better Sex,* published by Random House and based on a sex therapy program by the author, Domeena Renshaw, MD. Most recent is the *AMA Complete Guide to Women's Health,* published in the fall of 1996 by Random House.

As the millennium nears, the AMA's publishing activities continue to keep pace with the march of science — both the science of medicine and the science of communications. The Association launched its own home page on the Internet in 1995, offering physicians and the public highlights from the publications, political information, an AIDS/HIV information center, and other features such as AMA Physician Select — which enables patients to locate by name, specialty, or geographic area any of the approximately 650,000 physicians licensed in the United States. The technology, with the potential of communicating to millions of patients and of sharing information with medical colleagues around the world, could not even have been dreamed of by *JAMA*'s founders 112 years earlier, but the mission remains the same: educating the profession and the public about medical science and health care issues.

http://www.ama-assn.org

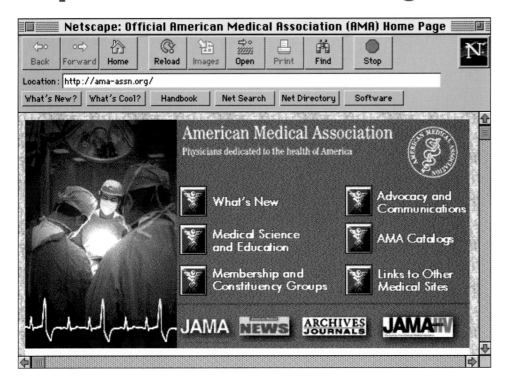

An AMA home page on the Internet reaches physicians and consumers alike around the world.

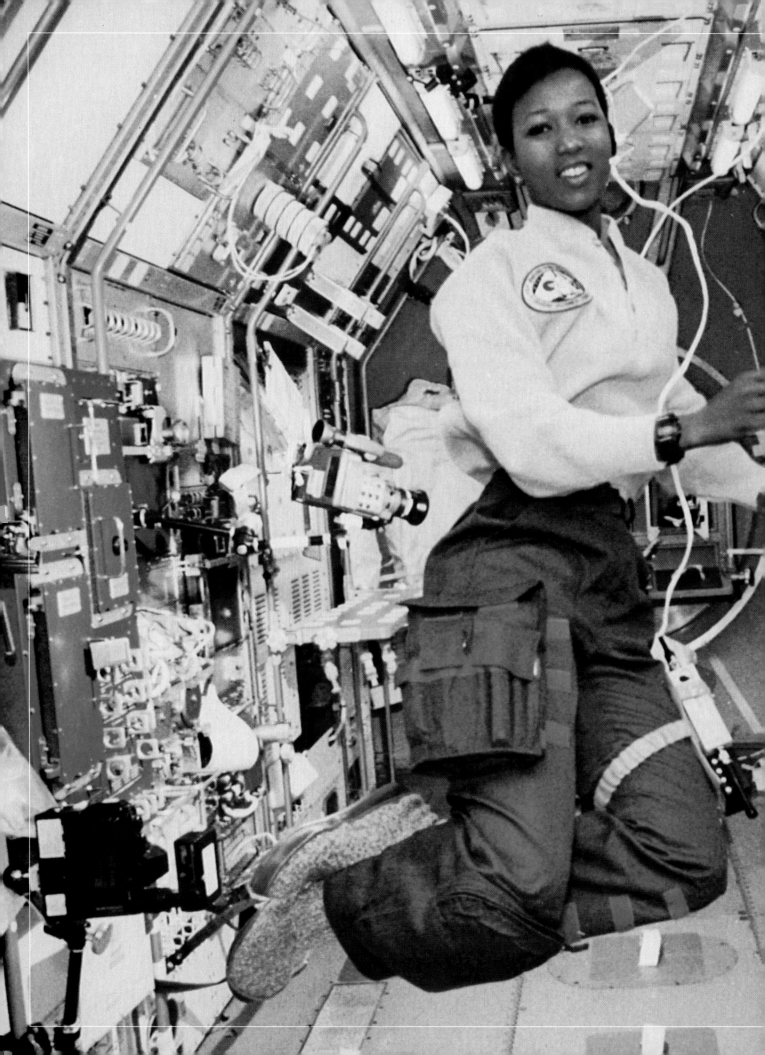

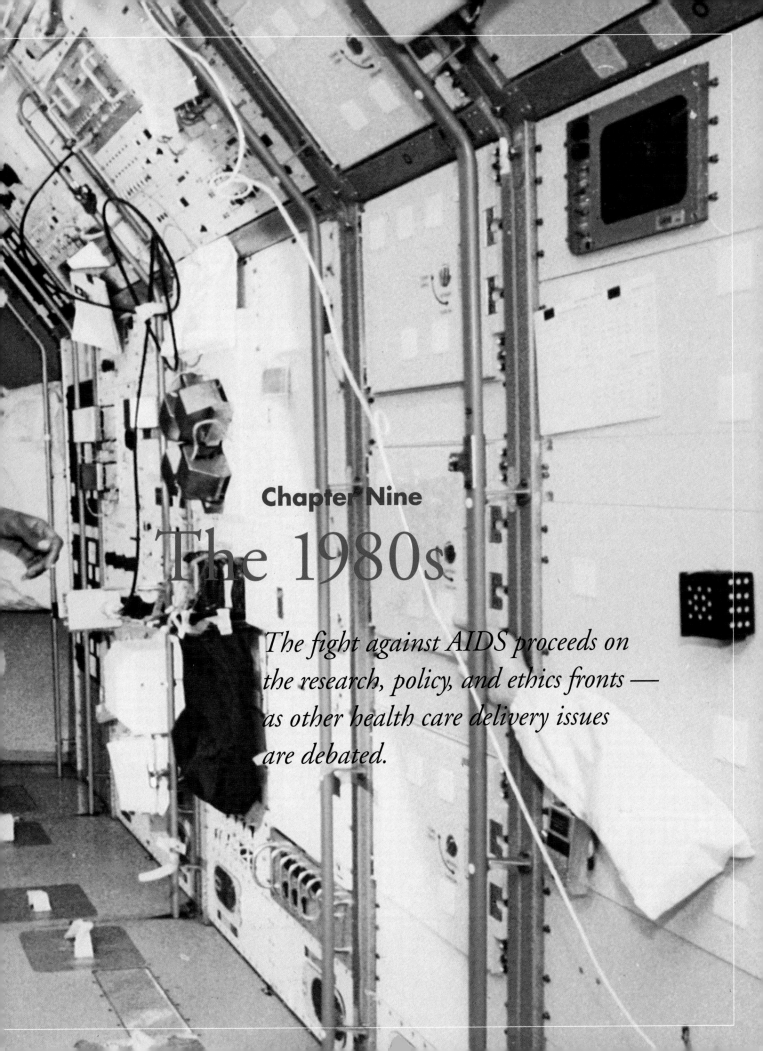

Chapter Nine

The 1980s

The fight against AIDS proceeds on the research, policy, and ethics fronts — as other health care delivery issues are debated.

The 1980s

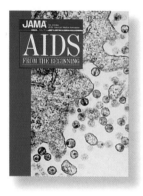

JAMA compiled its AIDS articles to assist scientists.

Overleaf: Astronaut Mae Jemison, MD, is weightless in space as she conducts her studies.

While the internal and external political battles that occupied much of the American Medical Association's time and energy in the 1960s and 1970s abated slightly in the next decade, major new challenges arose.

American Medical News, in an end-of-the-decade issue, called it "a decade of momentous change, of traditions shattered" and concluded, "Never have the challenges been greater, the pressures more intense, on the healing profession." The 1980s, the *News* went on, "saw the assimilation of technological advances once only imagined, while a deadly epidemic spread, resistant to the best ideas of medical science's finest minds. Advances in technique and equipment enhanced the power of physicians to defeat disease, while government intervention eroded physicians' authority over their practices. MDs achieved unprecedented levels of skill, yet found themselves repeatedly accused of malpractice and blamed for chilling the physician-patient relationship. The focus of care moved out of the hospitals, and the patient population steadily aged, compelling a reorientation of physicians' perspectives. Ethical dilemmas demanded of doctors the wisdom of the philosopher, while economic exigencies required sophisticated business expertise."

The most significant clinical challenge surfaced in 1981, with a little-publicized announcement by scientists in Los Angeles of a new and fatal disease:

acquired immunodeficiency syndrome. The profession and the public did not immediately recognize the impact of this discovery, but within a year it was clear that a major public health problem had developed.

In 1983, the AMA Council on Scientific Affairs summed up the situation in these words:

> *"The US population, particularly the homosexual male community, is presently frightened, and the medical community is baffled by the sexually transmitted disease known as acquired immune deficiency syndrome (AIDS). The advent of this disorder has ominous implications. More than 40% of those infected are dead within a year. Concern first developed when a June 1981 issue of* Morbidity and Mortality Weekly Report *(MMWR) revealed a number of cases of* Pneumocystis carinii *pneumonia (PCP) in formerly healthy homosexual males. Victims of this pneumonia are usually immunosuppressed. This MMWR also reported 26 cases of Kaposi's sarcoma in homosexual males. Although there is a reported high incidence of Kaposi's sarcoma in Uganda, the usual incidence of this disease in the United States is 1 in 10 million annually, predominantly in elderly men.*
>
> *"Other less common manifestations of AIDS include extensive varicella zoster, nocardiosis, cryptosporidia (an intestinal protozoal disease once recognized only in cattle and sheep), thrombocytopenia, histiocytic lymphomas, cryptococcus infections, toxoplasmosis, bladder and rectal cancers, atypical mycobacterial and* Mycobacterium avium-intracellulare *infections.*
>
> *"In June 1981, CDC began compiling statistics on AIDS. Since then, it has struck 788 people in the United States and 57 abroad, killing 295. Victims of AIDS thus far include four groups: male homosexuals (75% of all cases), IV drug abusers, Haitian immigrants, hemophiliacs, and five children in New Jersey."*

By the time the AMA House of Delegates reconvened in December of 1983, the Council had assembled an ad hoc advisory panel on AIDS and had developed basic guidelines for physicians who encountered patients with AIDS.

AMA responds to AIDS with clinical, ethical, and policy initiatives

As time progressed, the AMA moved ahead to develop policies that served as the basis for federal guidelines covering many AIDS situations, including confidentiality of testing, HIV-infected health care workers, contact tracing and partner notification, maternal screening and treatment, and many others. The 1996 *AMA Policy Compendium* contains 25 pages on AIDS and HIV infections, including some 70 separate policy statements.

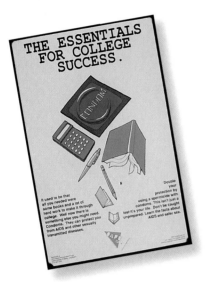

This public health poster from California State University/Long Beach focuses on condoms.

In December 1987, the Council on Ethical and Judicial Affairs addressed some of the issues stemming from the AIDS epidemic. Wrote the council: "The tradition of the American Medical Association, since its organization in 1847, is that: 'When an epidemic prevails, a physician must continue his labors without regard to the risk to his own health.' (*Principles of Medical Ethics,* 1847, 1903, 1912, 1947, 1955)." The Council called on physicians to preserve that heritage in these words: "A person who is afflicted with AIDS needs competent, compassionate treatment. Neither those who have the disease nor those who have been infected with the virus should be subjected to discrimination based on fear or prejudice, least of all by members of the health care community."

Throughout the decade, the AMA continued to involve itself in the public policy debate. It took a stand against most mandatory testing for antibodies to HIV (while recommending testing for pregnant women). It lent legal support to three Florida children who had been expelled from school because they were infected with HIV, and to a California teacher removed from classroom work after being diagnosed with AIDS. In 1987, the US Supreme Court supported the AMA and a host of other *amici* in *School Board of Nassau County v Gene H. Arline.* That case involved a Florida teacher fired after three bouts with tuberculosis. The key legal issue, which would eventually be applied to many AIDS cases, was whether such a contagious disease could be construed as a "handicap" under section 504 of the Americans With Disabilities Act.

A chronology of the late 1980s further demonstrates the AMA involvement in the war on AIDS:

- In 1985, the AMA called for expanded AIDS research and for additional government funding for such research.

- In 1986, the AMA opposed acts of discrimination against AIDS patients and legislative proposals that might lead to such discrimination or that would endanger patient-physician confidentiality. The AMA also developed and distributed professional guidelines for a physician's personal, clinical, and public conduct regarding AIDS.

- In 1987, the AMA urged development of an AIDS public awareness and information program and outlined a comprehensive approach for preventing and controlling the disease.

- In 1988, the AMA published and distributed 420,000 copies of *HIV Blood Test Counseling: AMA Physician Guidelines* and established an AMA Office of HIV/AIDS.

- In 1989, the AMA reiterated physicians' ethical responsibility to treat HIV patients whose condition is within the physicians' realm of confidence, and recommended that confidential testing be readily available to anyone.

- In 1990, the AMA published *HIV Early Care: AMA Physician Guidelines* and distributed copies to 350,000 physicians.

This AIDS poster featured hemophiliac AIDS patient Ryan White, who became a national symbol against discrimination.

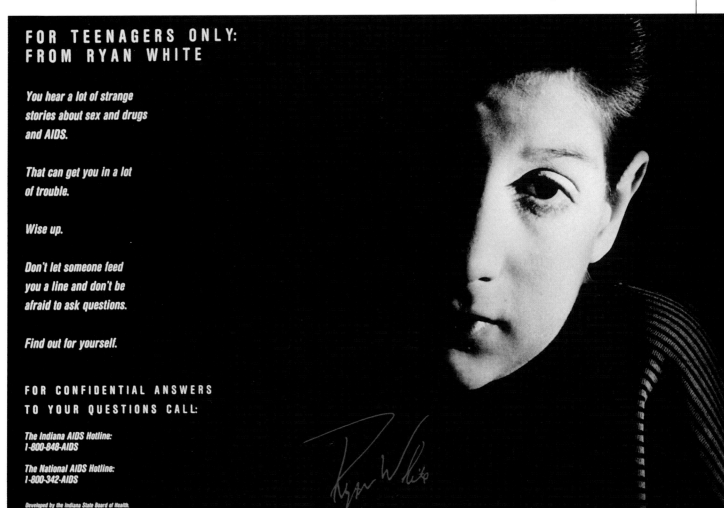

FOR TEENAGERS ONLY:
FROM RYAN WHITE

You hear a lot of strange stories about sex and drugs and AIDS.

That can get you in a lot of trouble.

Wise up.

Don't let someone feed you a line and don't be afraid to ask questions.

Find out for yourself.

FOR CONFIDENTIAL ANSWERS
TO YOUR QUESTIONS CALL:

The Indiana AIDS Hotline:
1-800-848-AIDS

The National AIDS Hotline:
1-800-342-AIDS

Developed by the Indiana State Board of Health.

As the decade ended, however, no real solution was in sight. An essay in *American Medical News* summed up the situation in these words:

"The inability of doctors to prevent mortality in AIDS patients reminded the profession of its role to care as well as cure. Growing reliance on technology had led to impersonal medical treatment, and observers described a crisis in the physician-patient relationship; studies found that patients filed malpractice suits less often because of bad outcomes than because of what they perceived as unfeeling treatment from physicians. At the decade's end, there was anecdotal evidence that some physicians were reorienting their approaches, spending more time with patients in an effort to recapture that trust."

Quality of life issues and ethics

Scientific advances also created several other ethical/legal issues during the 1980s. The "right to die" was pushed into the forefront by litigation in numerous states. The AMA Council on Ethical and Judicial Affairs responded with an opinion in 1986 that withholding of artificial nutrition from patients terminal or beyond doubt in a permanent coma was not unethical when done in consultation with the family. The opinion was welcomed and was cited within a year in rulings by appellate courts in California, Florida, and Arizona, in Massachusetts' highest courts, and by trial courts in New Jersey and California.

By 1988, the pendulum had swung the other way. In a widely publicized case, the Missouri Supreme Court refused to authorize the feeding tube withdrawal from 31-year-old Nancy Cruzan, who had been in a persistent vegetative state for some 5 years after an auto accident.

At the other end of the life cycle, so-called Baby Doe cases also took the spotlight in the 1980s, revolving around whether treatment can be withheld from severely handicapped newborns. The US Supreme Court in 1986 overturned federal regulations requiring treatment, but the issue remains today.

Also in the 1980s, the AMA took aim at a long-standing public health problem: tobacco and smoking. In 1983, the AMA issued a call for a smoke-free society by the year 2000 — still an Association goal. Another highlight was at the December 1985 meeting of the House of Delegates in Washington, DC. A Board of Trustees report called for a total ban on the advertising of tobacco products — the Association's strongest antismoking position up to that time. Congress was not in session, and the Washington media flocked to the AMA session. That same year, the AMA also supported legislation to ban smoking on public transportation, which was later enacted.

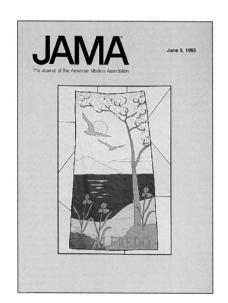

JAMA
The Journal of the American Medical Association
June 9, 1993

This detail from the AIDS quilt graced a *JAMA* cover in 1993.

Changes in the profession, changes in the Association

Changes in the entire fabric of the medical profession were under way in the 1980s as well. AMA President Harrison L. Rogers, MD, summed up the situation in his 1986 presidential address:

> *"Perfectly competent, conscientious doctors are practicing in solo or small partnership offices, being paid a fee for each service. Doctors who are just as competent and just as conscientious are practicing in shopping centers. They are salaried employees of hospitals and other institutions. They are members, whether by contract or by salary, of health maintenance organizations. They are participants in preferred provider organizations, negotiating their fees with a management service rather than with the individual patient. They are in large medical groups of single or multiple specialties. They are practicing in hospitals which have turned some of their rooms or floors into hotels and which have Wendy's or McDonald's in their lobbies to help their financial situation. They are in joint business ventures with hospitals, competing directly with other hospitals and with other physicians. And all of them, whatever their practice form, are trying to learn how to take care of patients who are unable to pay for everything they need because their insurance coverage is limited or because their government program has been cut back, or simply because they do not have insurance."*

A decade later, of course, Dr Rogers' remarks are still valid. The AMA, medical societies, and physicians are still grappling with the profound changes.

The 1980s also saw a major transition in the staff leadership of the AMA. James S. Todd, MD, thrust into the spotlight through his success as chair of the 1980 ad hoc Committee on Medical Ethics, had been elected to

For all of medicine, change abounded, and the AMA rose to the challenge of providing leadership.

the Board of Trustees. Five years later, Executive Vice President James H. Sammons, MD, tapped Dr Todd to be his principal deputy.

As executive vice president, Dr Sammons had become one of the most powerful individuals in the health care world. He was a frequent witness before Congressional committees and appeared regularly on public forums

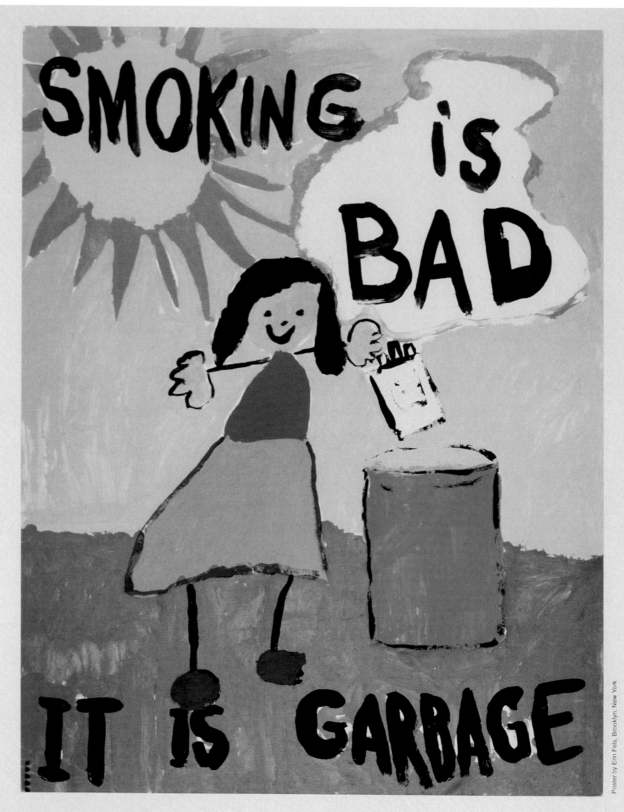

Poster by Erin Fels, Brooklyn, New York

SmokeLess States
Statewide Tobacco Prevention and Control

all over the country. Blunt and outspoken, he won the respect of friends and foes alike for his knowledge of and insight on health care issues and legislation. While politics and legislation were his first love, he played a major role in many of the Association's public health initiatives, particularly in the AIDS area.

Since taking over the financially floundering organization in 1974, Dr Sammons had also focused his energies on the AMA's bottom line. He had instituted many managerial reforms and business strategies that had placed the organization on a solid financial footing. He was a leader in the development of the AMA Washington office building at 1101 Vermont, which opened in 1982, and throughout much of the 1980s he pursued his dream of a new Chicago headquarters for the Association. After discussions with several developers and builders, the AMA struck a deal with the John Buck Company to occupy the lower 17 floors of a new 32-story building to be built at 515 N State St, across the street from the long-time headquarters at 535 N Dearborn.

Construction was well under way in 1989 when a Chicago newspaper published a series of articles alleging that Dr Sammons had inappropriately authorized two financial transactions that had worked to the advantage of three AMA senior staff members. A subsequent inquiry by the Board of Trustees and outside legal counsel determined that Dr Sammons had indeed acted inappropriately, although he had not personally benefited from any of the transactions. Dr Sammons, who had been scheduled to retire early in 1991, chose to step down in the spring of 1990, to be succeeded by Dr Todd.

Appearing for the first time as the executive vice president at the June 1990 meeting of the House of Delegates, Dr Todd set out at once to heal the wounds created by the Sammons controversy. "I have a vision for the AMA," Dr Todd told the delegates, "...a vision of you as champions of professionalism; demonstrating to all that we care for the least fortunate; that we will not accept less than the best for our patients and that in this

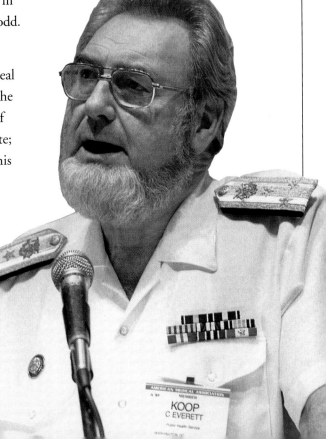

Surgeon General C. Everett Koop, MD, was an ally of AMA's public health efforts.

Facing page: This poster is part of the AMA's campaign for a smoke-free society by the year 2000.

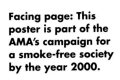

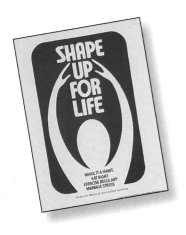

The AMA Alliance continues to stress public health themes, including the importance of exercise.

very real political world we must be accountable, we must be responsible and we must be responsive as we lead in charting the future of health care in this country."

Proposing new health care reforms

Coincidentally, that meeting of the House of Delegates came shortly after the AMA had unveiled its Health Access America proposal, which would be the cornerstone of the organization's health system reform activities for the next several years. Health Access America identified several categories of medical care expenditures over which physicians exert little control and proposed solutions to mitigate those expenditures. The following were key elements:

- **Professional liability reforms to minimize the need for defensive medicine.**

- **Changing the tax treatment of employee health benefits to reward individuals for making economical health insurance choices.**

- **Repealing mandated benefits laws.**

- **Developing practice parameters to define a range of acceptable treatment options.**

- **Reforming Medicare to ensure its financial viability.**

This framework placed the AMA in a strong political position as the decade ended. The 1980s had seen economics-driven changes that had significantly altered the landscape of health care. As costs rose and the elderly population grew in numbers, the federal government in 1983 had introduced prospective payments based on diagnosis-related groups, in effect capping hospitals' Medicare reimbursement. Private insurers followed suit with other reimbursement controls. Almost overnight, utilization review, preapproval of admission, second opinions for surgery, and other cost controls had become a part of almost every physician's practice. The trend away from private practice and into groups and health plans began to pick up steam.

At the same time, clinical medicine was advancing on many fronts. Magnetic resonance imaging was introduced in 1982 and became an essential feature of every hospital. There was laser surgery, multiorgan transplants, genetic engineering, and much more — all of it expensive. Also expensive was the increased ability to prolong life, even in the absence of any hope of recovery.

The escalation of health care costs (and the efforts of major employers to hold down their insurance premiums) and the increasing political and media interest in health system reform made a congressional push inevitable. Health Access America gave the AMA its own talking points and enabled medicine to claim a "seat at the table" in Washington when President Clinton launched his reform movement in 1993. It was a culmination of some 3 decades in which the Association had gone from a passive participant to a major player in the political arena.

AMA works for quality care and **liability reform as health care delivery** *undergoes major changes.*

Despite many changes, clinical training and care were still delivered at the bedside.

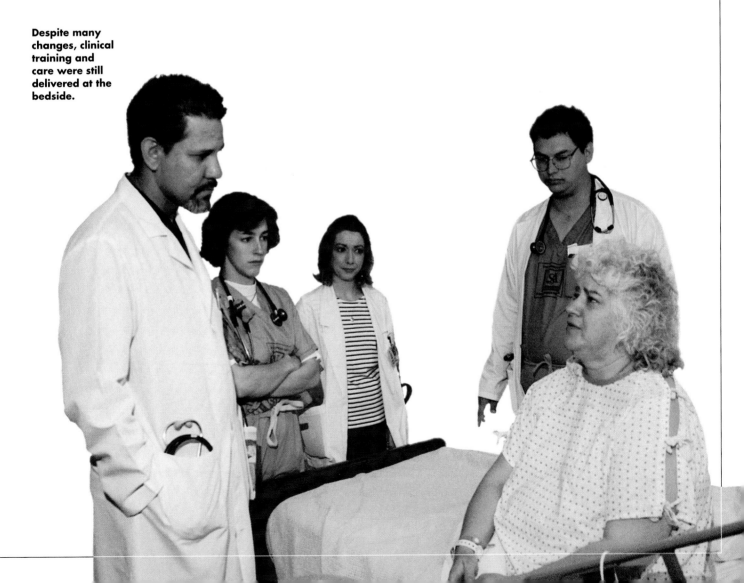

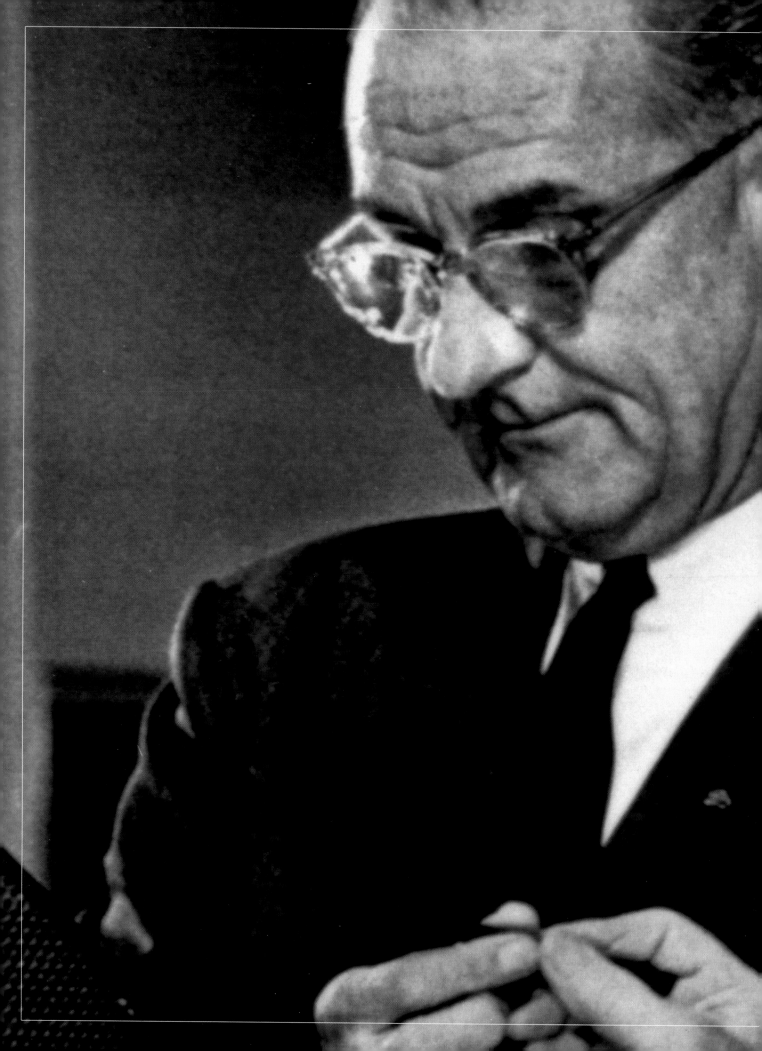

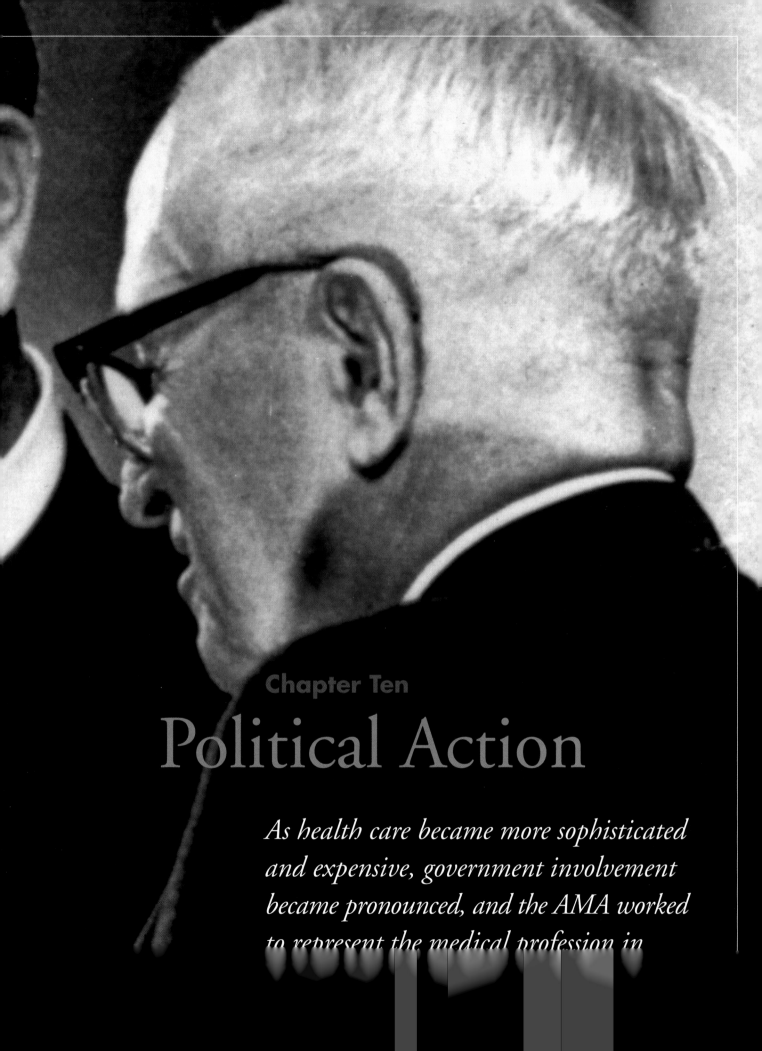

Chapter Ten
Political Action

As health care became more sophisticated and expensive, government involvement became pronounced, and the AMA worked to represent the medical profession in

Political Action

10

Throughout the first century of its existence, the American Medical Association was a reluctant participant in national politics. The organization's founders concentrated on education, ethics, and medical science. As the world changed — technologically, economically, socially, and politically — a point was reached when medicine had no choice but to speak out on behalf of patients and physicians in national public policy debates.

That point probably came at the time when World War II was winding down. The United States had just endured the Great Depression and the biggest war of all time, and the time was ripe for political upheaval. Even before the war, President Roosevelt had toyed with the idea of incorporating some health coverage into the Social Security program, but he was reluctant to endanger passage of that measure with the fight he knew would ensue over national health care.

Perhaps the turning point was the introduction of the Wagner-Murray-Dingell bill in 1943. That bill, introduced just 4 days before the AMA House of Delegates met, proposed a compulsory system of medical and hospital insurance for every individual (and dependents) covered by Social Security. It would have included a fee schedule for physicians' compensation. The bill's chief sponsor, Sen Robert Wagner (D-NY), insisted the measure was proposed for "legislative study and consideration."

Overleaf: President Lyndon Johnson presented former President Harry Truman the pen used to sign Medicare card No. 1 in 1966.

The AMA thought differently. At the House of Delegates meeting, a series of resolutions recommended some mechanism for expanding the AMA's presence in Washington.

This sentiment was far from unanimous, however. There were many defenders of the organization's traditional role, including General Manager Olin West, MD. He warned the delegates of the legal and political perils of turning the American Medical Association into a trade organization and insisted "that the AMA has no excuse for existence except as a scientific and educational organization." He was overruled by the delegates, however: the House voted to establish a Washington office and a new, powerful Council on Medical Service and Public Relations.

While the AMA was digesting this change, much of the battle against the Wagner-Murray-Dingell bill was carried out by the National Physicians' Committee, which was not a part of the AMA but which was led by two former AMA presidents and several former trustees. This organization raised money from industry sources and from contributions by individual physicians, and spent nearly a million dollars from 1940 to 1945 denouncing nationalized medical care legislation. One brochure was titled "Do You Want Your Own Doctor or a Job Holder?" and featured Sir Luke Fildes' painting, *The Doctor.* (The National Physicians' Committee's strident techniques eventually disenchanted many physicians; the group disbanded in 1951.)

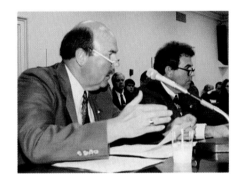

AMA is a frequent participant in Congressional hearings. Trustee William E. Jacott, MD, testified at this hearing in 1996.

With the pressures of the war, the 1943 Wagner-Murray-Dingell bill did not go anywhere. But shortly after the war's end, President Truman entered the fray, endorsing every American's "right of adequate medical care and the opportunity to achieve and enjoy good health." A new version of the Wagner-Murray-Dingell bill was introduced, and the AMA had a fight on its hands. The British National Health Act, socializing British medicine, was passed in 1946; several state legislatures also considered compulsory insurance schemes. Among them was California, where the state medical association hired the political advisory organization of Whitaker and Baxter to fend off legislation endorsed by Gov Earl Warren. The legislation failed by one vote in the California Assembly.

The drive for the Wagner-Murray-Dingell bill ran out of steam after extensive Congressional hearings in 1946, and the Republicans captured Congress in that fall's elections. Coupled with the AMA-backed drive for voluntary health insurance through Blue Cross and Blue Shield, it appeared that the issue of national health insurance had come to a dead end. President Truman's upset victory over Thomas E. Dewey in the 1948 election changed all that.

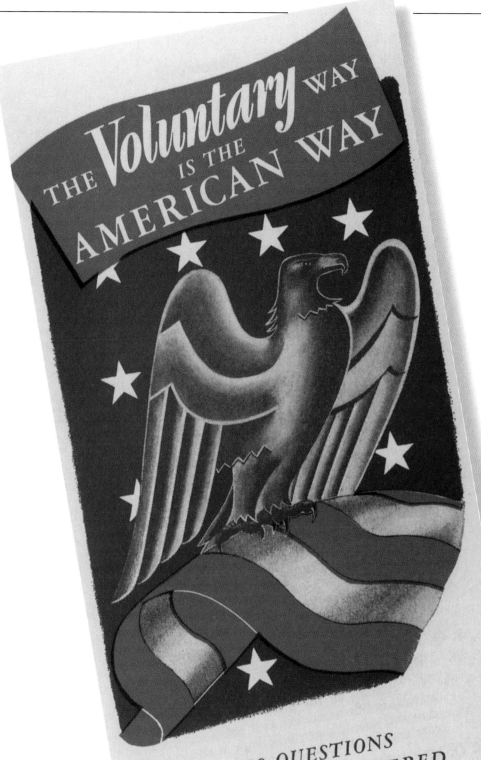

THE **Voluntary** WAY IS THE **AMERICAN WAY**

50 QUESTIONS
YOU WANT ANSWERED
on

**COMPULSORY
HEALTH INSURANCE**
Versus

Health...the American Way

This brochure was part of the AMA's campaign against President Truman's national health insurance plan.

The AMA response to health insurance legislation in the Truman and Eisenhower years

Truman had campaigned on his "Fair Deal" platform, which featured social benefits including compulsory national health insurance. The AMA responded immediately, moving to expand the Washington office, assessing its members $25 each in 1949, and hiring the California political consultants Whitaker and Baxter to provide advice on the coming battle.

Clem Whitaker and Leone Baxter — husband and wife — had helped Earl Warren become governor of California in 1942 and had helped the California Medical Association defeat Warren's compulsory insurance proposal 3 years later. They were in the forefront of the political movement to mobilize grassroots support for (or against) a specific proposal or individual. They cloaked their message in emotional, patriotic terms that might seem unsophisticated today — Fildes' *The Doctor* painting appeared everywhere, as did the flag — but there was no questioning their zeal and effectiveness.

Their campaign called for a rapid expansion of voluntary insurance through Blue Cross and Blue Shield, with the ringing slogan "The Voluntary Way Is the American Way." But the main thrust of the Whitaker-Baxter campaign was to convince legislators that all sorts of local organizations were backing the AMA's position on the issue. At the June 1949 meeting of the AMA House of Delegates, Whitaker and Baxter reported that their firm had made direct contact with, and stated the AMA's case to, 4500 Lions clubs, 2300 Rotary clubs, and 1500 Kiwanis clubs; with 1300 Carnegie libraries, 900 college libraries, and 8000 public libraries; with 130,000 dentists and druggists; with 12,000 trade associations and 2700 chambers of commerce; and with 14,000 school principals and superintendents.

Grassroots political activity has become a key element of AMA's political strategy. At the 1996 National Leadership Conference, medical society representatives from Georgia (left) and Florida (right) met with their representatives in Congress.

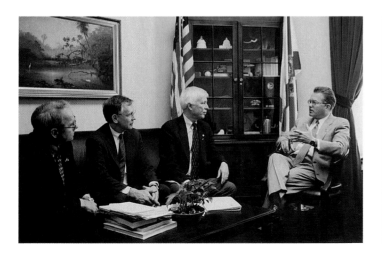

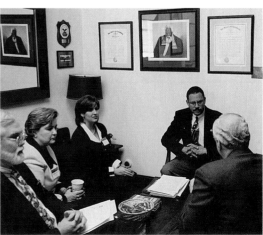

The campaign was a success. Widespread opposition, including that of many Southern Democrats in Congress, doomed Truman's legislation. For the AMA, the event was a watershed. Some 65% of AMA members had paid the 1949 assessment (bringing in some $2.3 million) and membership climbed from 140,000 in 1948 to nearly 148,000 in 1950. But there were many physicians — both in positions of power and in the grassroots — who felt the AMA was straying from its proper course as a scientific and professional organization. However, the growing public, media, and governmental interest and involvement in health care activities had made it impossible to divorce medicine and politics. As things turned out decades later, the American Medical Association would prove it was possible to combine political activism with all the best features of a professional medical organization: scientific information, standard setting, patient advocacy, and ethics.

The Eisenhower presidency from 1953 to 1960 did provide a respite from the immediate legislative pressures. But in 1957, Aime Forand, a Connecticut Democratic congressman, had introduced a labor-backed national health insurance proposal that returned the issue to the spotlight and drew the sponsorship of a young Democratic senator from Massachusetts, John F. Kennedy. At the same time, individual physicians in some regions of the country were entering the political arena, forming local committees and working for the election of candidates whose views matched theirs.

These groups gave impetus to the American Medical Association's decision to launch the American Medical Political Action Committee (AMPAC). Another push came from the formation of the Committee on Political Action (COPE) by the AFL-CIO; this was probably the first national committee of its type. AMA Executive Vice President F. J. L. Blasingame, MD, supported the concept of a PAC for medicine, and his deputy, Ernest B. Howard, MD, was a staunch advocate. In the wake of John F. Kennedy's election to the presidency in 1960, the Board of Trustees in early 1961 approved the formation of AMPAC.

AMPAC develops into a major political presence

AMPAC would go on to become one of medicine's most successful activities. There were several bumps in the road, however, including a bitter dispute over AMPAC's role in the ouster of Dr Blasingame as executive vice president in 1968 and the selection of James H. Sammons, MD — a onetime AMPAC board chair — as the AMA's CEO in 1974.

The AMA has become a shaper and **staunch advocate of legislation addressing** *the nation's health care needs.*

At the same time, AMPAC was widely admired by professional politicians as one of the most effective organizations in the national arena. Its masterstroke was to build from the bottom up rather than from the top down, as did the governors of labor's COPE. AMPAC developed a structure that relied on state-organized PACs, making it one of the first to foster a genuine grassroots political action committee. Within 15 months, 45 states had functioning medical PACs, bringing physicians and allies at the local level into political activities. A training program was established to prepare potential campaign workers for candidate support. Educational materials, including training films and pamphlets, were targeted for physicians and spouses — through the Woman's Auxiliary to the AMA — to bring them into campaigns. They were drilled in such basics as voter registration and precinct organization. They also became involved in AMPAC's pioneering work in studies in voter polling, research, and analysis. Thus, when successful candidates arrived on Capitol Hill, they were well aware of the AMA.

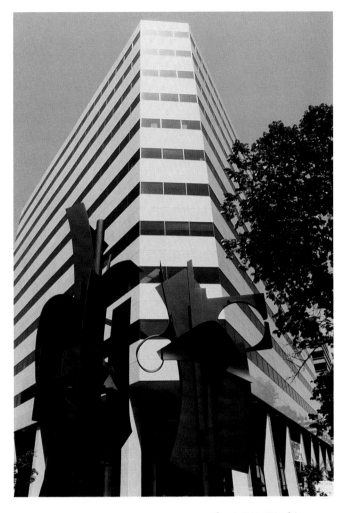

The AMA's Washington office, dedicated in 1982, was another milestone in AMA's political growth.

Since its founding, AMPAC has remained a leader within the political community, using its visionary tactics and innovative political activities to assist friends of medicine in their quest for public office. It consistently has been at the forefront of the development of new methods to express political support, being one of the first to develop independent expenditure ads used in key races when it was clear AMPAC could make a difference. Its grassroots network today, aided by sophisticated electronic systems, is on the leading edge of political involvement. Others have been impressed, and sometimes shaken, by the effectiveness of the AMA's PAC. This movement represented a departure from previous reliance on aggressive public relations campaigns and lobbying alone. AMPAC Board Chair Frank Coleman, MD, said in 1965: "The solution…to keeping politics out of medicine no longer lies in asking Congress to act wisely; the solution lies in helping to elect a wise Congress." A beneficial side effect: numerous conservatively oriented interest groups followed AMPAC's lead, demolishing what had been labor's monopoly in this field. The impact of this movement is still being felt nearly 4 decades later.

Social policy and the courts

"Creating Health Policy in the Courts," a 1991 paper from the AMA Office of the General Counsel, summarized the AMA's legal efforts from 1989 to 1991 in cases affecting the physician-patient relationship and the health of the public. The AMA proceeds on this assumption:

"Medicine is unique — a very special profession with goals and standards that set it apart from other businesses and occupations. The courts consistently need to be made aware of this fact so that the law and its interpretation do not erode the profession's distinct place in our society."

The AMA's legal intervention continues to the present day. In what type of cases does the AMA intervene on behalf of the profession and the public? The issues include patient rights, managed care, antitrust laws, professional liability, government regulation of the profession, and many others.

In recent years, several cases involved the patient-physician relationship. In *Cruzan v Director of the Missouri Department of Health,* the US Supreme Court cited the AMA's brief in a 1990 decision upholding the right of patients to have artificial life supports withdrawn. In so-called Baby Doe litigation, the AMA in 1984 joined a successful challenge to federal regulations that would have required reporting of suspected discrimination by physicians against impaired newborns. And in the Association's sesquicentennial year, it is expected to be heavily involved as the US Supreme Court considers assisted suicide.

An earlier case with broad implications was *School Board of Nassau County v Gene H. Arline,* in which the Supreme Court in 1987 upheld the AMA's contention that an individual with an infections disease is "handicapped" under terms of the Rehabilitation Act. The 1983 case dealt with a tuberculosis patient, but the decision also affects AIDS patients.

More recently, the AMA has joined with more than 30 national medical specialty societies to form the AMA/Specialty Society Medical Liability project, which is supporting federal tort reform legislation.

Frank D. Campion, a long-time AMA employee during this period, provides this analysis in his 1984 book, *The AMA and U.S. Health Policy Since 1940*:

> "*It is inaccurate to say that the AMA leaders of the 1950s and early 1960s were ignorant of the way things worked in Washington. They knew perfectly well what sort of pressures were brought to bear on legislation and, as a matter of fact, the AMA seldom hesitated to exert pressures of its own. There was certainly no shyness about stating the AMA position on matters of policy either to the public or to congressional leaders.*
>
> "*The trouble was that AMA leaders, up until the late 1960s, came on as crusaders, as fierce, unyielding believers in principles that could not be compromised. Admirable as such strength of conviction may be, it puts the holder at a disadvantage, especially where disputes are settled by parliamentary methods. The crusader is always throwing down the gauntlet and offering his adversary a hard choice: a fight to the death or unconditional surrender. The crusader makes it all but impossible for a legislature — especially a legislature responsive to a diversity of interests — to follow his lead.*
>
> "*But after 1965, when the AMA suffered a dramatic rout in the legislative struggle over Medicare, a new generation of leaders slowly came to power. Although these physicians held much the same beliefs as their predecessors, their style was different. They avoided getting locked into rigid positions, for they were not crusaders but pragmatists. They had a more realistic understanding of the political process; they were better equipped to operate within it. And, because AMPAC served as a training ground for many of these physicians, that may well be the most enduring of AMPAC's achievements.*"

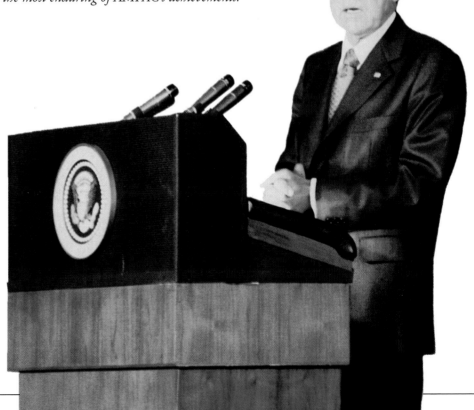

President Richard Nixon addressed AMA delegates in June 1971.

The national health insurance debate — from the 1960s to the 1990s

AMPAC's early years were politically difficult ones for medicine, however. President Kennedy had thrown his wholehearted support behind the King-Anderson bill for medical care for seniors as a part of Social Security. The AMA had countered with Eldercare, a voluntary program for the needy elderly. The initial result was a victory for medicine, as the Senate in 1962 turned down the King-Anderson bill. But President Kennedy's assassination, Lyndon Johnson's ascension, and his landslide victory in 1964 (carrying a huge Democratic congressional majority on his coattails) made the 1965 passage of Medicare inevitable.

Beyond that, many people were viewing Medicare as only the first step toward a complete national health insurance program for all. This possibility had motivated some AMA leaders to develop their own mechanism for financing care. A key figure was Russell B. Roth, MD, then a member of the Council on Medical Service and later speaker of the House of Delegates and president of the AMA in 1973. A witty, articulate urologist from upstate New York, Dr Roth in the early 1960s took the lead in the development of a detailed legislative proposal that would have enabled the AMA to offer a viable alternative to Medicare. The Board of Trustees and the House of Delegates eventually refused to back the proposal, opting instead for all-out opposition and prompting Dr Roth to muse that the organization was in a "profound state of autohypnosis."

The idea did not go away, however, and after detailed studies by the Council on Medical Service, the Council on Legislative Activities, and various other groups, the House of Delegates in June 1968 gave its approval to the Comprehensive Health Care Insurance bill. Introduced in Congress in 1969 as Medicredit, it was based on retaining Medicare, voluntary participation, and continued reliance on the existing system. It would have used federal income tax revenues to subsidize private health insurance for everyone except Medicare beneficiaries. The subsidies would be based on demonstrated need.

This sent a message to Congress: the AMA was recognizing the economic problems in the health care system and was proposing a solution, rather than opposing change. And change was contained in a 1970 bill backed by labor and introduced by Sen Edward Kennedy that would have federalized the entire health system. President Nixon countered with his own proposal,

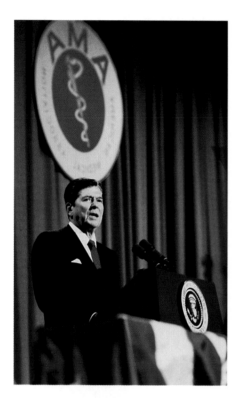

President Ronald Reagan spoke to the AMA Annual Meeting in 1983, warning of the rising cost of care.

including mandated employer coverage, state aid for low-income and high-risk patients, and Medicare improvements. In all, the early 1970s saw about a dozen major health care bills before Congress and lobbyists of all persuasions swarming over Capitol Hill.

The AMA was well represented and persuasive. Records show the AMA spent $114,000 on lobbying in 1971, and, Campion recalls, the lobbyists "found themselves beneficiaries of the preceding nine years of work done by AMPAC. Mindful of medicine's support back home at election time, many congressmen and their staff assistants lent the AMA an attentive ear."

Eventually, nothing would come of any of this batch of legislation; the divisions among the various factions were too wide. The most serious move toward national health insurance in the 1970s came in August 1974, weeks after President Nixon's resignation. President Ford, in his August 12 inaugural address, urged Congress to "sit down and sweat out a sound compromise… Why don't we write a good health bill on the statute books before this Congress adjourns?" Stimulated, the Republicans, labor and Sen Kennedy, and the influential chairman of the House Ways and Means Committee, Wilbur Mills of Arkansas, sat down and drew up a compromise bill including mandated employer-employee–paid health insurance, catastrophic coverage, and a federalized Medicaid program. Mills then met with AMA leaders, who voiced adamant opposition to the plan's Social Security financing features.

When Mills called his committee to order on August 20, he appeared to have a workable coalition in support of his proposal. When the committee began to vote, however, things fell apart. After a disheartening series of tie votes, one-vote victories, and an 11–7 vote to make part of the plan voluntary, Mills adjourned the mark-up session for the day. The next morning, he ran up the white flag. "I've never tried harder on anything in my life than to bring about a consensus on this bill," he said. "But we don't have it. I'm not going to go before the House with a national health insurance bill approved by any 13–12 vote."

That anticlimactic moment marked the end of any serious discussion of a national health insurance program until President Clinton's 1994 attempt. It did not stop the American Medical Association from continued emphasis on political activity, both in Washington, DC, and at the grassroots level.

The Washington effort was particularly significant. The AMA's presence in Washington began in the 1940s as a one-person office staffed by Joseph Lawrence, MD. During the Truman administration and throughout the 1950s,

Gradually, AMA's posture moved from **opposition to advocating its own solutions** *to national problems.*

the Washington office grew gradually to some 15 employees, including lobbyists and media relations staff. But during the Kennedy years of the early 1960s, the AMA began establishing itself as a major Washington presence. The AMA moved to a new office building on Farragut Square South, doubled the size of the staff, and expanded its efforts in all sectors of the Capitol.

Sen Edward Kennedy's late 1960s–early 1970s campaign for national health insurance, coupled with the AMA's growing activism and Congress' growing interest in health care activities, stimulated more growth and another move to new quarters, this time at 1776 K St NW. But the AMA's establishment as a major player on the Washington scene was emphasized in 1982 when the AMA's Washington staff moved into the top two stories of a new AMA-owned office building at 1101 Vermont Ave. (The building has since been sold — at a significant profit — but the AMA's 65-member Washington staff still occupies $2^{1}/_{2}$ floors.)

The AMA and the White House

The AMA's Washington presence was also furthered by appearances at its meetings by two US Presidents. Richard M. Nixon chose the AMA's 1971 Annual Meeting in Atlantic City to ask for medicine's support in his new war on drugs — "an all-out battle against the drug menace." A key provision in Nixon's proposal was the recognition of methadone's role as a maintenance drug rather than a withdrawal drug and the development of methadone clinics to help addicts lead more active lives. Nixon also spoke out against a national health insurance proposal being supported by Sen Edward Kennedy, warning that it "would exact a very high price from our people in terms of dollars and cents. But it would exact an even higher price in terms of the quality of American medicine."

The AMA responded enthusiastically, just as it did in 1983 when President Ronald Reagan came to Chicago to address the House of Delegates. Reagan did issue a warning about the growing costs of health care, citing an inflation rate $2^{1}/_{2}$ times that of the overall economy. "It is high time," he said, "we put health care costs under the knife and cut away the waste and inefficiency. The growth in medical costs is malignant and must be removed for the continued health of the American people." Reagan proposed three specific reforms — prospective payment, catastrophic coverage under Medicare (later enacted and then repealed), and capping tax-free health insurance benefits.

The next resident of the White House to address the AMA House of Delegates was not a president but a first lady. Hillary Rodham Clinton came to Chicago in the summer of 1994, in the midst of an eventually

At the beginning of the debate over President Clinton's health system reform legislation, First Lady Hillary Rodham Clinton brought the Administration's message to the AMA House of Delegates in June 1993.

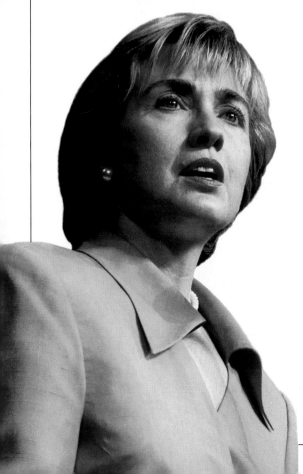

fruitless campaign to enact comprehensive health system reform. She spoke warmly of the contributions of the medical profession, and the House of Delegates responded with an ovation. Two years later, the Republicans had seized control of both houses of Congress, and the new speaker of the House of Representatives, Newt Gingrich of Georgia, had asked the AMA for its Medicare recommendations. The AMA responded with a detailed proposal — based on its Health Access America document — for transforming the Medicare program along with other reforms, and Gingrich appeared via a closed-circuit TV hookup to thank the physicians for their efforts. At the December meeting in 1995, Gingrich appeared in person, urging medicine's support for Republican-backed reforms, including measures to address Medicare's impending fiscal crisis.

That support was forthcoming, but White House vetoes and government shutdowns blamed on Congress torpedoed any changes in Medicare. With Medicare reform off the table, Congress and the Administration turned to incremental health care reforms long advocated by the AMA. President Clinton announced creation of a National Commission to ensure patient protections in health insurance plans. The FDA announced various controls over tobacco use, based on its addictive character. Reforms in antitrust rules, patient protection legislation, fraud and abuse provisions, and mental health parity became the focus of AMA advocacy. Soon there was no mistaking the AMA's impact on Washington legislative activities. With members of the vast Physicians Grassroots Network contacting their legislators, and its aggressive presence on the Hill, the AMA successfully pushed the FTC's publication of revised rules governing the formation of physician-controlled health networks, argued for passage of laws ensuring reasonable lengths of stay for maternity patients, supported revised fraud and abuse legislation, and initiated the first steps leading to insurance parity for psychiatric patients. The breadth and depth of physician concern, guided by the AMA and AMPAC, were communicated to lawmakers. Medicine's message was heard.

The American Medical Association, persuaded by societal changes to become a political advocate, not only had done so, but also in the process had risen to the top as a national example of effective political advocacy. It moved from what many considered a "just say no" political position to a tireless and pragmatic advocate for policy positions it developed itself. At age 150, the AMA had become a major force in the development of the nation's health policy. This would be demonstrated convincingly as the 20th century approached its close.

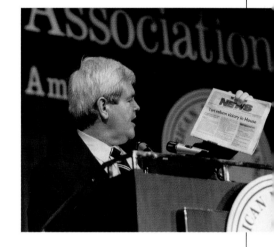

House Speaker Newt Gingrich (R–Ga) brought the Republicans' plan for health system reform to AMA delegates at the 1995 Annual and Interim meetings.

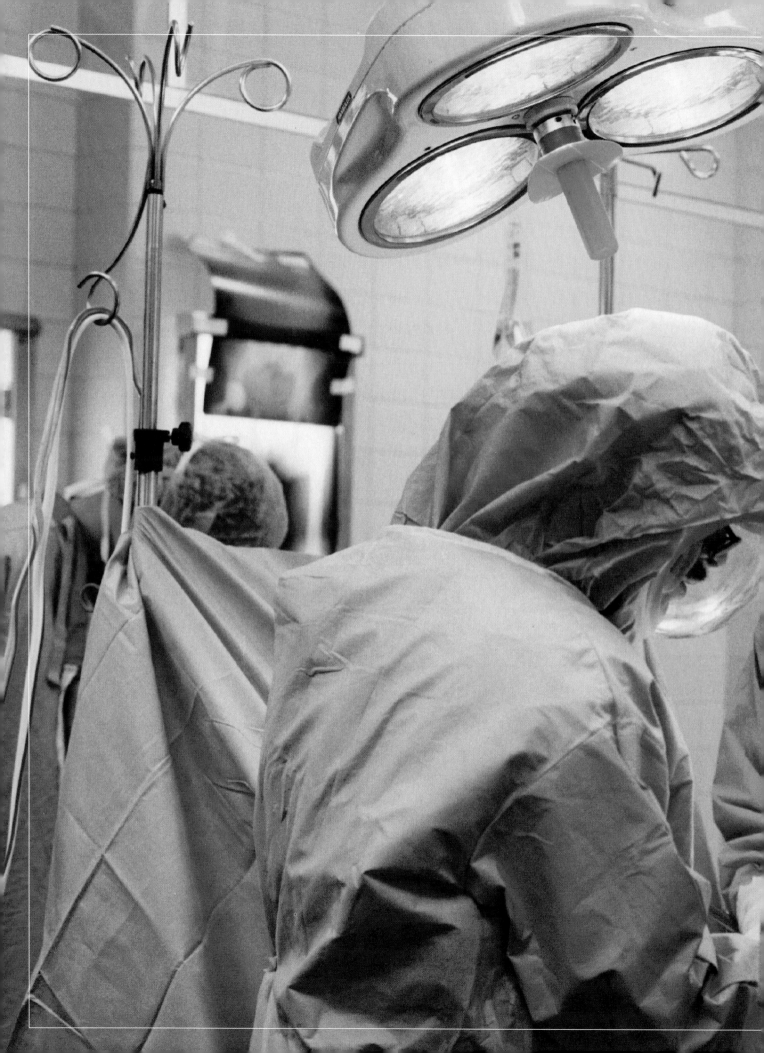

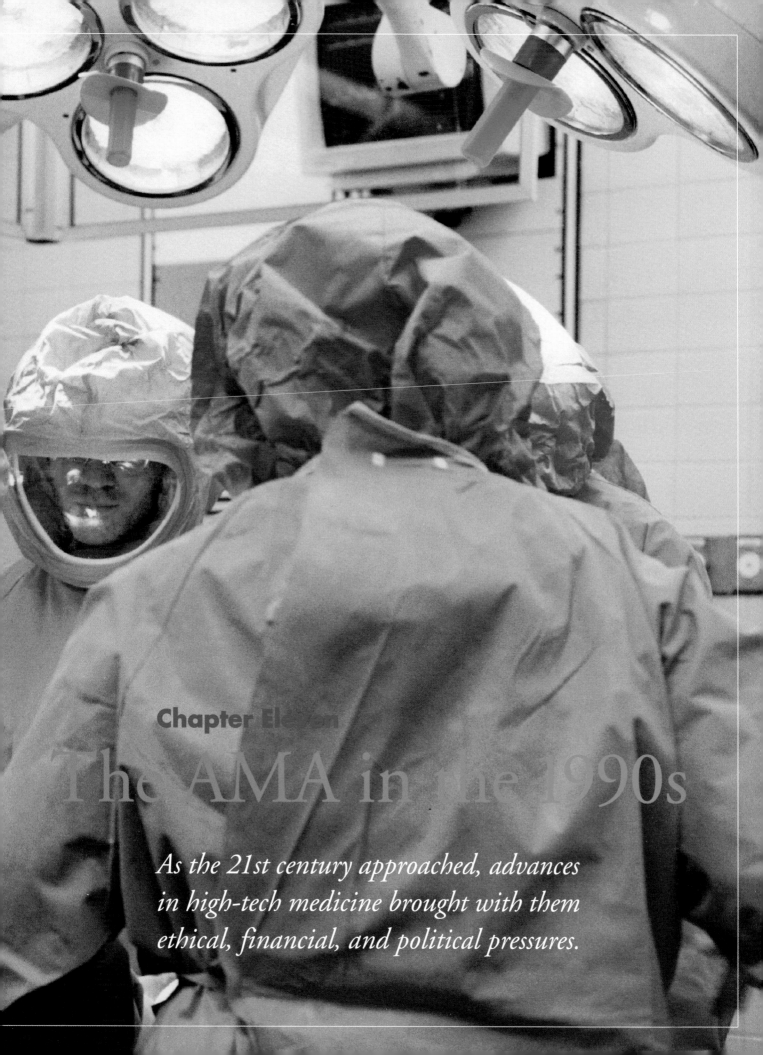

Chapter Eleven

The AMA in the 1990s

*As the 21st century approached, advances
in high-tech medicine brought with them
ethical, financial, and political pressures.*

The AMA in the 1990s

With its sesquicentennial just around the corner and with the 21st century looming, the American Medical Association entered the 1990s with a full head of steam. In the last half of the 20th century, America was undergoing a transition from a largely segregated society to one in which women and individuals from minority groups are regarded as legitimate candidates for the office of Presidency of the United States. As an American institution, the AMA is proud of its own uniqueness; but at the same time, the AMA is also proud that it has reflected the cultural changes occurring in the larger American society. For example, in 1985 Lonnie R. Bristow, MD, was elected the first African-American trustee and, in 1995, the first African-American president of the AMA. Nancy W. Dickey, MD, was elected first woman trustee of the AMA and went on to become Board chair in 1996. Palma E. Formica, MD, was the first international medical graduate to be elected to the Board. Also, in 1996, Regina Benjamin, MD, an African-American woman, was elected to the Young Physicians' slot on the Board. The AMA has become a leader in painting the new American canvas.

On many fronts, things were looking up at the start of the 1990s. The AMA had just moved into sparkling new headquarters offices. Medical student and resident trustees were taking an active role. Executive Vice President James S. Todd, MD, was in the early stages of what would be a distinguished 6-year term. His eventual successor, P. John Seward, MD, was serving on the AMA Board of Trustees, a group he would later chair.

Overleaf: Infection control is a key component of surgery today.

Dr Bristow, looking back at a long career in organized medicine, expresses pride in the AMA's record of growth in addressing discrimination. As the country has changed, so has the medical profession, and so has the American Medical Association, he states. He points to the wide range of AMA policies that not only oppose discrimination within the profession but also espouse the human rights of patients, regardless of race, gender, or medical condition. The evolution of the AMA reflects the growing diversity in the leadership of all medical organizations, notes Dr Bristow, himself a former president of the American Society of Internal Medicine. He adds, "The AMA can honestly say that it is a part of the solution to *all* problems that significantly affect the nation's health and welfare."

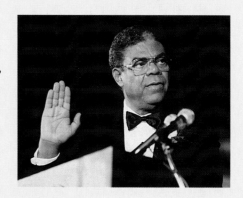

Lonnie R. Bristow, MD, became the AMA's first African-American president in 1995.

However, there would be no honeymoon for medicine. The AIDS epidemic was continuing unabated, with no vaccine or cure in sight. The rising costs of health care — brought about in large part by technological advances — were creating strong new pressures to control costs. One solution that created nearly as many problems as it solved was managed care. Advances in technology also were raising serious ethical issues as society grappled with how resources should be allocated. *American Medical News* addressed this problem in a special issue with the theme "Who Lives, Who Dies? Who Decides?" and summed up the dilemma in these words:

> *"In recent years a technological imperative — a mandate to use all available means to preserve life* because *these means exist — has driven medicine to focus enormous resources on the critically ill....Stormie Jones and Nancy Cruzan both are beneficiaries of the technological imperative. Jones, the recipient of the first heart-lung transplant, died last November [1990] at age 13. She had enjoyed several extra years of life — years for which her friends and family are grateful. In contrast, the family of Cruzan, who is in a persistent vegetative state, waged a series of court battles to have her nutritional support discontinued. The Cruzans are not grateful for what medical science can do."*

The rise of managed care and new attempts at health system reform

Some of these problems would be inextricably linked with the trend toward managed care. As the decade wore on, some health care plans, eyeing the bottom line, sought ways to limit the amount and types of care made available to terminally ill patients. The combination of factors would make end of life issues the topic of major ethical debates as the decade continued. As he left office, Dr Todd summed up the problem in these words: "I was chair of the committee that rewrote the Principles of Medical Ethics in 1978–1980. We were roundly criticized for talking about physicians' responsibility to society. But we were ahead of our time. No longer is it possible for physicians to take into account only the individual patient. The physician must remain the advocate of that patient, but must temper advocacy with reality. If you look only at the individual patient, you say, 'I will do everything possible for this patient — I don't know whether it will work or not, but I'll do it.' And you start doing heart transplants on 80-year-olds."

With Republican President George Bush in office as the decade began, the prospects for major national health legislation seemed remote. The election of Bill Clinton to the presidency in 1992 gave new impetus to national health legislation. Supported by a massive publicity drive to convince the public that health care was one of the nation's major problems, President Clinton chose first lady Hillary Rodham Clinton to develop a sweeping reform proposal. After several months of meetings with advisers, the White House came forward in 1993 with a complex proposal that, if accepted whole by Congress, would have affected virtually every patient and physician. Hillary Clinton came to the AMA Annual Meeting in 1993 to attempt to enlist medicine's support for the White House proposal. Her address to the delegates was largely conciliatory and upbeat, focusing in the main on problems with the existing system that affected physicians as well as patients. She emphasized that the White House task force had "benefited so much from what you have already done, and from the involvement of many of you around the country." She stated that "we are not talking just about reforming the way we finance health care. We are not talking about the particulars of how we deliver health care. We are talking about creating a new sense of community and caring in this country — in which we once again value your contribution, value the dignity of all people."

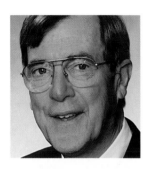
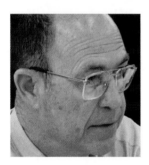
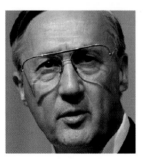

AMA's leadership as its sesquicentennial neared included (from top) President Daniel Johnson, Jr, MD; Board Vice Chair Thomas R. Reardon, MD; and President-Elect Percy Wootton, MD.

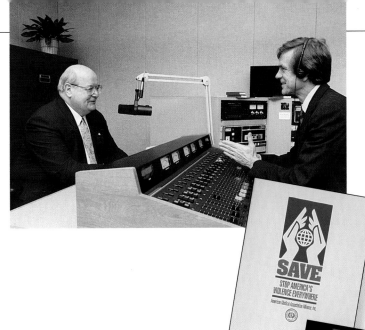

Robert E. McAfee, MD, AMA president in 1994–1995, is interviewed for American Medical Radio News. Dr McAfee has been a leading spokesperson against family violence.

Two or 3 decades earlier, the AMA would have reflexively — and vigorously — opposed any such entreaties. This time, armed with political savvy and the existing recommendations of Health Access America, the AMA remained neutral — supporting elements not only of the White House proposal but also of other reform legislation that matched its own policies, opposing those that were contrary to it, and emphasizing all the while that there were serious access and delivery problems that needed to be addressed.

In the long run, the Clinton proposal sank without ever getting close to a final vote in either house of Congress. By the time members of Congress went home for the 1994 off-year elections, the Clinton legislation had been abandoned, a victim of its own cumbersome bureaucratic and big-government proposals and of partisan politics. However, the failure of Clinton and the Democratic-controlled Congress to act on health care was seen by many observers as a contributing factor in the Republicans' sweep into control of both houses of Congress that fall.

As the AMA had warned, one problem that truly needed solving was the financing of Medicare. In early 1995, ominous predictions about the long-range fiscal prognosis for the program motivated the new Republican speaker of the House of Representatives, Newt Gingrich of Georgia, to call on the AMA — and several other organizations — for suggestions for reform. The AMA was prepared; a document entitled "Transforming Medicare" already was in place — again based largely on Health Access America — and many of the AMA's suggestions wound up being incorporated into the Republican-drafted Medicare legislation. Speaker Gingrich appeared on closed-circuit TV to thank delegates at the 1995 Annual Meeting, and hopes were high for passage of legislation. This time, however, it was the Republicans' plan that fell victim to partisan politics and election-year wrangling, leaving the nation heading into the end of the century with the financial future of its largest health program still up in the air.

151

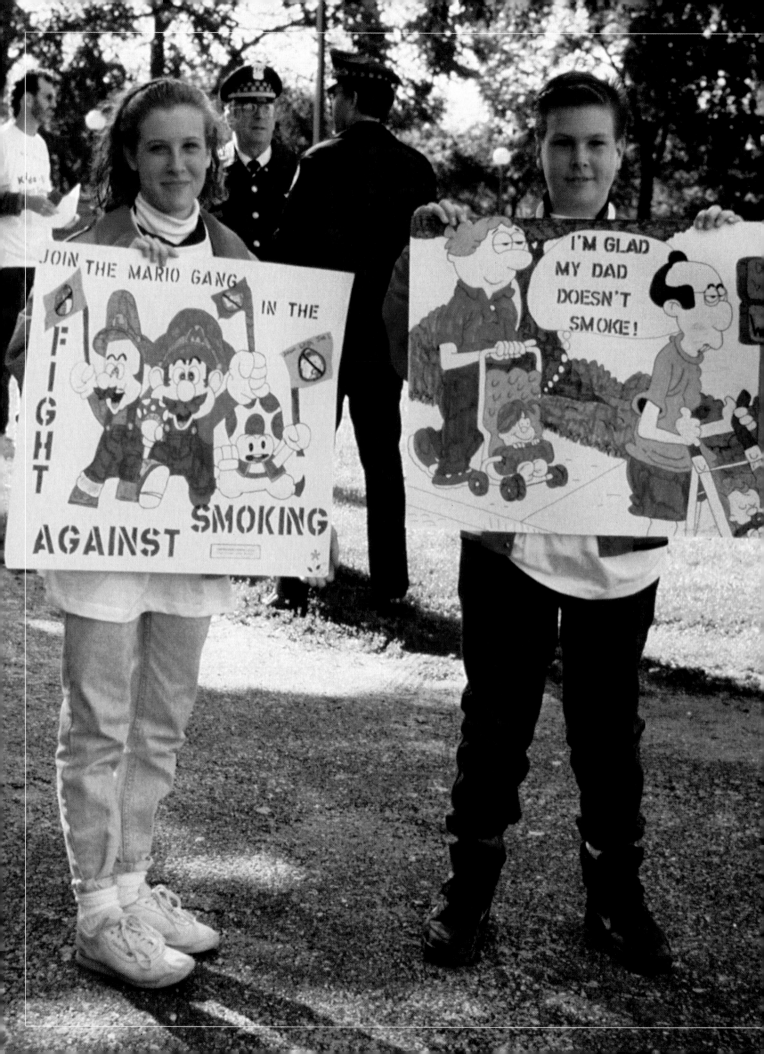

Campaigns for public health issues

A side effect of Washington's reluctance to take on national health legislation was that it enabled the AMA to direct its efforts and resources into significant public health issues. One of those was violence. Working in conjunction with the AMA Alliance and its chapters across the country, the AMA launched a major campaign targeting all types of violence and placing particular focus on domestic violence. Publication in *JAMA* of an annual violence report card received widespread media and public attention. The "Physicians' Campaign Against Family Violence" involved thousands of physicians all over the country.

In the '90s, advocacy efforts focused on public health issues, **particularly smoking, substance abuse, violence, and end of life care.**

The Alliance, working locally with many county medical societies, developed the "SAVE" program (Stop America's Violence Everywhere). By 1996, more than 55,000 physician spouses were involved in efforts in some 650 communities to bring together physicians, the public, and local officials in rallies, vigils, and forums. A community guidebook was being readied for publication in 1996, and a series of regional conferences were planned to help develop coordinated community responses to family violence.

Robert McAfee, MD, AMA's president in 1994–1995, became one of the nation's most articulate and dedicated speakers for the antiviolence activities. Addressing physician audiences, he often described a personal

The campaign for a smoke-free society also took to the streets; AMA sponsored this protest against "Joe Camel."

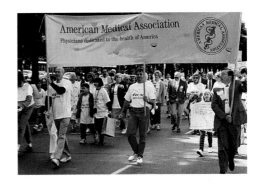

Facing page: The AMA's anti-tobacco program reached out to young people such as these participants in a poster contest.

consciousness-raising experience that occurred during an appearance on a panel discussion on domestic violence. Chatting with another physician on the panel, Dr McAfee remarked, "I understand you treat battered wives." "Yes, doctor," was the reply, "and so do you." In 1995, the AMA issued the first physician guidelines on sexual assault.

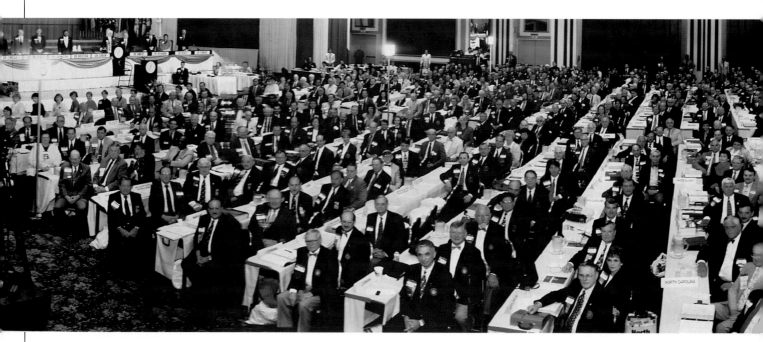

At the 1996 Annual Meeting, members of the House of Delegates look forward to the 150th birthday of the AMA in 1997.

The war on tobacco products was another major AMA campaign in the 1990s. Building on previous efforts, the AMA attacked on several fronts. *JAMA* published a set of documents depicting the tobacco industry's efforts to conceal from the public and Congress the data about the health problems of smoking. A precedent-setting editorial signed by the entire AMA Board of Trustees supported the attack. The AMA called on investors — including mutual funds — to get rid of their stocks in tobacco companies. Targeting children, the AMA took on "Joe Camel" and readied its own antismoking cartoon character, "The Extinguisher," to raise young people's consciousness about the hazards of tobacco use.

Also targeted in the 1990s was alcohol abuse. The Robert Wood Johnson Foundation provided the AMA's Division of Health Science with $20 million for programs to reduce alcohol-related problems among underage youth as well as binge drinking among college students. At the other end of the spectrum, the AMA sent to 110,000 primary care physicians a set of guidelines on alcoholism in the elderly, calling attention to a long-neglected problem that affects thousands of families.

Ethical and practice issues also were in the spotlight as the 1990s progressed. Responding to the rising costs of care, insurers and businesses sought new mechanisms for controlling expenditures. This led to the boom in managed care, which was anathema to some physicians, panacea for others. For all, however, it led to difficult ethical situations as physicians came under

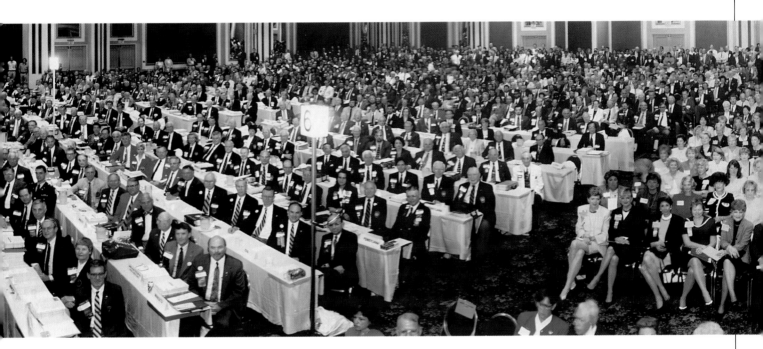

increasing pressure from their health plans to hold down costs. This trend led to a highly visible and successful AMA campaign against so-called gag clauses, which proscribed physician disclosure of some costly treatment options not covered by the health plan. In January 1996, *JAMA* published a precedent-setting opinion from the Council on Ethical and Judicial Affairs, "Ethical Issues in Managed Care." These guidelines affirm that physicians will not allow the patient-physician relationship to be altered in any system of health care delivery. At the same time, the AMA published a series of resource documents to help physicians in dealing with managed care issues.

Another major ethical topic revolved around end of life issues. Despite pressure from some consumer groups and in the face of some adverse court decisions, the AMA continued its adamant opposition to physician-assisted suicide, which the House of Delegates reaffirmed in 1996. At the same time, the AMA collaborated with the American Bar Association and the American Association of Retired Persons to develop and publish a model advance-directive handbook, "Shape Your Health Care Future."

AIDS continued to be a major problem for all of medicine as well. In addition to the daunting search for a successful vaccine or therapy, issues of patient testing, confidentiality, and disclosure continued to occupy ethicists and policymakers as the decade wore on. Meanwhile, the AMA developed an HIV/STD prevention kit to help patients reduce high-risk sexual behavior. Subsequently, in 1996, the AMA published a series of physician guidelines to help them address AIDS/HIV issues.

Sesquicentennial and reorganization — looking toward the future

As the sesquicentennial neared, the House of Delegates in June 1996 gave its final stamp of approval to a major overhaul of the AMA's structure of governance. The proposal, designed to expand specialty society participation in the AMA and to provide a more cohesive and unified medical profession, won approval after some 3 years of effort by a consortium chaired by the tireless Joseph T. Painter, MD. It was Dr Painter who more than 2 decades earlier had chaired the committee that had steered the AMA out of the worst

Facing page: Today, the AMA's headquarters staff occupies the first 16 floors of this contemporary building at 515 N State St, Chicago.

As the first woman chair of the Board of Trustees of the AMA, Nancy W. Dickey, MD, looks to the future of the AMA in its next 150 years. "What keeps the AMA vibrant is the continuing dedication of the men and women of medicine who — each and every day — turn the AMA's legacy of leadership and healing into concerned care for our patients."

As a practicing physician, Dr Dickey sees ethics as a key issue that will affect physicians and patients alike. She sees the new AMA Ethics Institute "as the ethical beacon for physicians working to keep up with changes in health care." Further, she views the American Medical Accreditation Program (AMAP) as a pace-setting drive to accredit physicians that will ensure quality care.

Futurologists are busy analyzing possible changes in medical science and health care in the next century, but Dr Dickey is confident that a rededication to the physician-patient relationship will be the cornerstone of all AMA members' commitment to their patients and their profession.

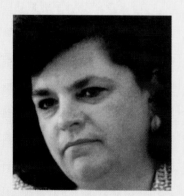

Nancy W. Dickey, MD, first woman Board chair.

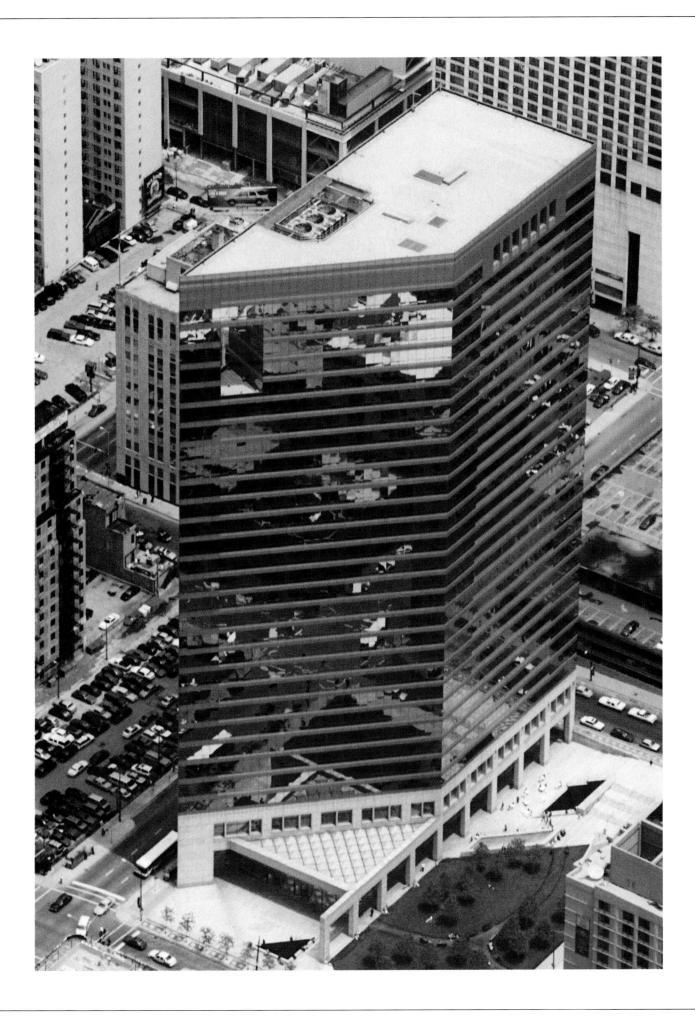

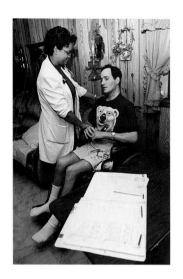

AMA Trustee Regina Benjamin, MD, makes a house call to a patient in rural Alabama.

financial crisis in its history. A Texas internist who had gone on to become AMA Board chair and president, Dr Painter saw the historic action — the biggest change in the AMA's organization since the House of Delegates was formed 95 years earlier — as "just the beginning of change." He added, "We're talking about a new federation, a different federation, one that includes all significant groups of physicians…We're building on the strengths of individual organizations at the same time we seek greater collaboration."

At that same 1996 meeting, the Association's new executive vice president, P. John Seward, MD, took note of the organization's upcoming sesquicentennial. When the AMA was founded, he pointed out, "It was a vast and different time. The railroad and telegraph had yet to network the country… Our population was barely 20 million…Physicians of every kind numbered less than 25,000. Formal medical societies were small in number and weak. Today, our population is pushing toward 300 million. Our profession is bursting with more than 700,000 physicians and medical students. The AMA recognizes 645 county, state and specialty medical societies, many of them big, well-organized and powerful both inside and outside."

Dr Seward continued:

"Much has changed in 150 years, or so it would seem. But a hard core of basic principles still forms the AMA's foundation. Principles like patient advocacy, ethics, education, professionalism, standard-setting, quality of care. These principles define who we are, what we do, what we stand for. Together, they form a value system that has bonded the men and women of American medicine into a coherent, cohesive professional organization, renowned for our service to patients and the public and respected for our staying power. We are more than just an American institution. We are an American icon, perceived as a leader, the protector of the patient-physician relationship and the voice of medicine."

The American Medical Association's founders, Dr Nathan Davis and his colleagues, lived in a different world, but they would undoubtedly nod in agreement at Dr Seward's words. The practice of medicine changes constantly and rapidly, and it would be folly to attempt to predict the environment for the AMA's bicentennial in 2047.

One constant will remain, however: virtually all of medicine will continue to be practiced one-on-one, physician to patient. The medical profession's commitment to this principle — putting the patient first — has been the foundation of the world's premier health care system. Whatever the future holds, this key element of medicine's proud heritage will remain.

Through 150 years of change, the **AMA's commitment to putting patients first** *has remained constant.*

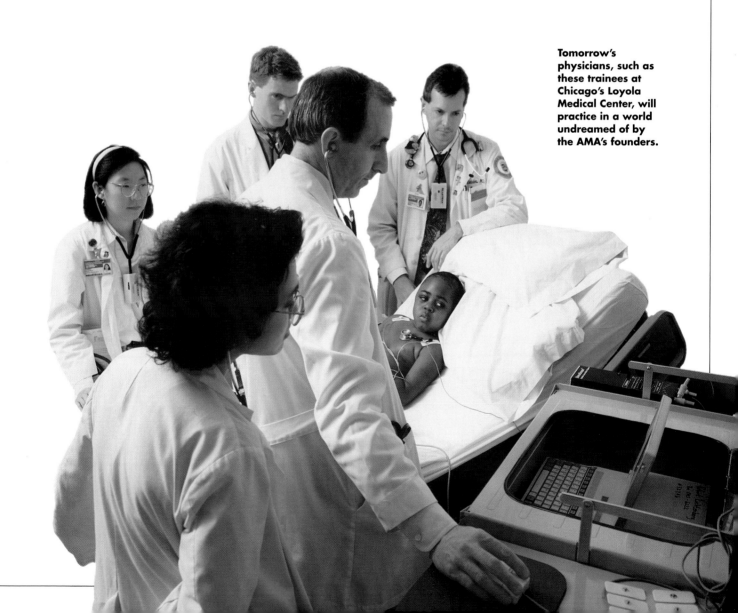

Tomorrow's physicians, such as these trainees at Chicago's Loyola Medical Center, will practice in a world undreamed of by the AMA's founders.

The American Medical Association: A Chronology **1847–1997**

1847

Founding of AMA at Academy of Natural Sciences in Philadelphia (Founder Nathan Davis)

AMA Committee on Medical Education appointed

AMA Code of Medical Ethics written and published

AMA sets first minimal standards for medical education

1848

AMA notes the dangers of universal traffic in secret remedies and patent medicine

1849

AMA establishes a board to analyze quack remedies and nostrums and to enlighten the public in regard to the nature and dangerous tendencies of such remedies

1858

AMA establishes Committee on Ethics

1868

AMA Committee on Ethics strongly advocates recognition of regularly educated and qualified female physicians

1869

Archives of Ophthalmology founded under title *Archives of Ophthalmology and Otology*

1870

AMA recommends that Congress pass a national system of quarantine regulations

1873

AMA Judicial Council founded to deal with ethical and constitutional controversies

1876

Sarah Hackett Stephenson becomes first woman member of AMA

AMA adopts a resolution promoting sanitary municipal water supplies and sewer systems

1882

Archives of Dermatology founded under title *Journal of Cutaneous Diseases*

1883

Journal of the American Medical Association founded; Nathan Davis is first editor

1884

AMA supports experimentation on animals as the most useful source of knowledge in medical practice

1897

AMA incorporated

1898

AMA Committee on Scientific Research is established to provide grants for fostering medical research

1899

AMA creates Committee on National Legislation to represent the Association's interest in Washington

AMA establishes Council on Exhibits to promote public health education

Dr George H. Simmons begins a 25-year appointment as editor of *JAMA* and develops the journal into an internationally recognized publication

AMA appoints a committee to report on the nature of tuberculosis, means of control, public education, and advisability of establishing national and state sanatoriums

AMA urges that local boards of health adopt laws requiring compulsory smallpox vaccination

1901

AMA reorganizes, creating the House of Delegates

1902

AMA acquires its first permanent headquarters in Chicago

1904

AMA establishes the Council on Medical Education to accelerate campaign to raise educational requirements for physicians

1905

AMA establishes Council on Pharmacy and Chemistry to set standards for drug manufacturing and advertising and fight the war on quack patent medicines and nostrum trade

AMA Council on Medical Education develops and publishes in *JAMA* minimum and ideal curriculum standards for medical schools

1906–1907

AMA Council on Medical Education inspects 160 medical schools and classifies them into three groups: A = acceptable; B = doubtful; and C = unacceptable

1906

AMA Council on Medical Education publishes directory of medical schools in the United States, detailing entrance requirements

AMA Chemical Laboratory is established to analyze nostrums and drugs submitted for AMA review (in the 1930s, leading to the AMA Seal of Acceptance)

AMA publishes first American Medical Directory listing over 128,000 licensed physicians in US and Canada

AMA membership exceeds 50,000

1908

Archives of Internal Medicine founded

1910

The Flexner Report, *Medical Education in the United States and Canada,* funded by the Carnegie Foundation and supported by the AMA, is published and facilitates new standards for medical schools. The report cites many diploma mills

AMA Council on Medical Education publishes the first edition of *Essentials of an Acceptable Medical College,* revised eight times in the next 41 years, to be superseded by the *Functions and Structure of a Modern Medical School*

1911

Archives of Pediatrics and Adolescent Medicine founded under title *American Journal of Diseases of Children*

1912

The Federation of State Medical Boards is established accepting AMA's rating of medical schools as authoritative

AMA approves a report of the standard methods for prevention and control of tuberculosis

1913

AMA establishes a "Propaganda Department" to gather and disseminate information concerning health fraud and quackery

1914

AMA Council on Medical Education sets standards for hospital internship programs and publishes first list of approved hospitals offering such programs

AMA adopts a resolution approving establishment of uniform milk standards and classification of milk

1915

AMA publishes favorable report on government-supported health care through sickness and accident insurance for employed individuals

1919

Archives of Neurology and Psychiatry founded

1920

AMA acquires *Journal of Cutaneous Diseases* and changes title to *Archives of Dermatology and Syphilology*

Archives of Surgery founded

AMA opposes compulsory health insurance through an August 1920 resolution by the House of Delegates

Council on Medical Education becomes Council on Medical Education and Hospitals

1922

Woman's Auxiliary to the AMA is organized to assist the AMA in its program for the advancement of medicine and public health

1923

Hygeia, the AMA's family health magazine, is founded

AMA adopts standards for medical specialty training

1924

Morris Fishbein begins 25-year tenure as editor of *JAMA* and *Hygeia*

The AMA begins radio broadcasts that bring health messages to the general public

1925

Archives of Otolaryngology — Head and Neck Surgery founded under title *Archives of Otolaryngology*

AMA Propaganda Department becomes Bureau of Investigation

1926

Archives of Pathology and Laboratory Medicine founded under title *Archives of Pathology*

1927

AMA Council on Medical Education and Hospitals publishes first list of hospitals approved for residency training

1929

AMA acquires *Archives of Ophthalmology*

AMA Council on Foods established as a subgroup of Council on Pharmacy and Chemistry

1930

AMA requests evaluative psychiatric services be made available to every criminal and juvenile court, and to correctional institutions

1931

AMA's Bureau of Medical Economics is established to study all economic matters affecting the medical profession

1934

Official recognition of specialty boards in medicine begins through collaborative efforts of the AMA Council on Medical Education and the Advisory Board for Medical Specialties (and later by its successor, the American Board of Medical Specialties)

1935

Social Security Act is approved. It does not include compulsory health insurance because of AMA influence

1936

AMA Council on Foods becomes Council on Foods & Nutrition; council offers AMA Seal of Acceptance to food manufacturers who pass advertising and content tests and who conform with Food and Drug Act; council encourages enriching milk with vitamin D to prevent rickets, and salt with iodine to prevent goiter

AMA membership exceeds 100,000

1937

AMA asks county medical societies to share the burden of caring for poor patients

1938

AMA Council on Foods and Nutrition publishes *The Normal Diet,* containing the first authoritative dietary recommendations for Americans

1940

Council on Pharmacy and Chemistry discontinues analysis of drugs and directs efforts to providing physicians with information on efficacy of dosage administration; encourages the advancement of new drugs by issuing development grants

1942

The AMA Council on Medical Education and the Association of American Medical Colleges establish the Liaison Committee on Medical Education to accredit programs leading to the MD degree

1943

AMA opens office in Washington, DC

AMA Council on Medical Service and Public Relations is established

1944

AMA receives a commendation from the Surgeon General for the radio series "Doctors at War," as an excellent service to the Medical Department of the US Army

1945

AMA recommends borderline limits to determine alcohol influence in the suspected drunken driver

1946

AMA begins television broadcasts that bring health messages to the general public

1947

AMA celebrates centennial of its founding

1948

AMA launches a campaign against President Truman's plan for national health insurance

1950

Hygeia becomes *Today's Health*

AMA Council on Medical Education, along with the Association of American Medical Colleges, develops and publishes a list of foreign medical schools with educational programs that meet AMA standards

1951

Joint Commission on Accreditation of Hospitals is formed by the American College of Surgeons, American College of Physicians, American Hospital Association, AMA, and the Canadian Medical Association

AMA endorses the principle of fluoridation of community water supplies

AMA Education and Research Foundation established to help medical schools meet expenses and to help medical students

1953

National Internship Matching Program is formally established

1954

AMA Council on Medical Education establishes the Internship Review Committee

First list of continuing education courses is published by AMA Council on Medical Education

AMA recommends equipping all automobiles with safety belts

AMA establishes Committee on Geriatrics to outline basic problems of aging and how to deal with them

1954–1955

Council on Foods & Nutrition discontinues Seal of Acceptance program and focuses efforts on providing nutritional information to the profession and the public

1955

Archives of Dermatology and Syphilology becomes *Archives of Dermatology*

AMA supports a 5-year program for states to improve mental health care

AMA approves extension of Water Pollution Act and programs to eliminate air pollution

1956

AMA declares alcoholism an illness

AMA Council on Pharmacy and Chemistry becomes Council on Drugs

1957

The AMA Council on Medical Education convenes discussions that lead to the formation of the Educational Council (now the Commission) for Foreign Medical Graduates

1958

American Medical Association News begins publication

1959

Archives of Neurology and Psychiatry splits to become two separate journals: *Archives of Neurology* and *Archives of General Psychiatry*

1960

AMA recommends a nationwide vaccination program against polio using the Sabin oral vaccine

AMA states that a blood alcohol level of 0.1% should be accepted as *prima facie* evidence of alcohol intoxication

AMA develops national policy on health care for older patients

AMA Archives is established to preserve AMA historical documents and serve as a resource center

1961

The American Medical Political Action Committee (AMPAC) is formed to represent physicians' and patients' interests in health care legislation

AMA takes responsibility for updating *Standard Classification of the Nomenclature of Disease*

AMA establishes Continuing Education Advisory Committee to develop standards and mechanisms for the evaluation and accreditation of all programs of continuing medical education

1962
Dr Edward Annis gives speech in Madison Square Garden, in response to President John F. Kennedy's speech on Medicare delivered in the same location

AMA publishes the first edition of the *Style Book;* this becomes the *American Medical Association Manual of Style* in 1989

AMA holds the first National Congress on Mental Health

AMA establishes Committee on Medicine and Religion to encourage communication between physicians and clergy on the most effective care of patients

1963
AMA publishes first edition of *Current Medical Terminology,* a system of preferred and supplementary terms and descriptors for diseases

AMA Council on Medical Education and Hospitals becomes Council on Medical Education

AMA establishes the Committee on Environmental Health

1964
AMA adopts a report on the hazards of cigarette smoking

1965
AMA scientific meeting has largest attendance and is referred to by the *New York Daily News* as the "Biggest Doc Bash Ever"

AMA adopts a statement recognizing the dangers of air pollution and provides a medical basis for governmental action

AMA holds the first of seven Western Hemisphere Nutrition Congresses

AMA News becomes weekly publication

AMA membership exceeds 200,000

1966
AMA publishes first edition of *Current Procedural Terminology (CPT),* a system of standardized terms for medical procedures used to facilitate documentation

AMA encourages physicians to promote exercise as a means to better health

1966–1975
AMA organizes and administers Vietnam Medical School Project

1967–1973
AMA coordinates Volunteer Physicians for Vietnam program

The United States Adopted Names Council is established to determine nonproprietary designations for chemical compounds

1968
AMA Physician's Recognition Award program is established, providing certificates to physicians who qualify by completing required amounts of continuing education

AMA adopts a statement on infant mortality with 14 recommendations for reducing the infant mortality rate in the US

1969
American Medical Association News becomes *AMNews*

1970
AMA urges the FAA to require all airlines to separate nonsmokers from smokers

AMA Center for Health Services Research and Development is established

AMA opens membership to osteopaths

1971
AMA creates Department of Field Service with 12 regional offices to provide on-site assistance to state and county offices

AMA publishes the first *Guides to the Evaluation of Permanent Impairment*

First edition of AMA *Drug Evaluations* published, a source of comparative evaluative information on drug therapy

AMA adopts report to Board of Trustees reviewing changes needed to increase the number of women physicians

1972
AMA opens membership to students and residents

AMA launches war on smoking, urging the government to reduce and control the use of tobacco products and supporting legislation prohibiting the disbursement of samples of tobacco

Liaison Committee on Graduate Medical Education established to accredit residency programs

1973
AMA urges physicians to cooperate in a national program to combat hypertension

1975
AMA establishes a National Commission on the cost of medical care

Woman's Auxiliary to the AMA becomes the AMA Auxiliary

AMA adopts resolution opposing sex discrimination in medical institutions

1976
AMA Section on Medical Schools established

AMA encourages handicapped access to public facilities

AMA endorses and encourages establishment of a permanent Office of Surgeon General of the US Public Health Service

1977
Liaison Committee on Continuing Medical Education established to accredit continuing medical education courses

AMA sponsors first meeting of the Resident Physicians Section

1978
AMA supports state legislation mandating the use of seat belts and other protective restraints for infants and children

AMA reorganizes House of Delegates to include representatives of national medical specialty societies

AMA develops national policy endorsing hospice care to enable the terminally ill to die in a more homelike environment

1980
AMA establishes the Medical Student Section

AMA launches the French edition of *JAMA,* the first of 28 international editions of the *Journal* established between 1980 and 1996

AMA holds first Health Reporting Conference

AMA Council on Medical Service issues a report on the impact of health maintenance organizations on quality, access, and costs of care

1981
AMA holds first annual Science Reporters Conference

Accreditation Council for Graduate Medical Education replaces Liaison Committee on Graduate Medical Education

AMA recommends that current studies on the effects of "Agent Orange" and dioxin be expanded and that all physicians be alerted to symptoms of exposure

Accreditation Committee for Continuing Medical Education replaces Liaison Committee on Continuing Medical Education

1982
George Lundberg begins serving as editor-in-chief of *JAMA* and Scientific Publications

AMA encourages each state medical society to seek and support legislation to raise the legal drinking age to 21

AMA Consumer Publishing program begins with the first edition of *AMA Family Medical Guide,* published by Random House

AMA initiates the Health Policy Agenda for the American People, with a 28-member steering committee representing various health, business, and consumer organizations (which led up to Health Access America)

AMA adopts resolution calling for increased representation among women and minority physicians

American Medical Radio News begins

1983
AMA organizes Hospital Medical Staff Section, later renamed Organized Medical Staff Section

AMA urges a smoke-free society by the year 2000

AMA membership exceeds 250,000

AMA and the Health Care Financing Administration (HCFA) sign an agreement requiring the use of CPT in federal programs for the reporting of physicians' services, as part of the administration's common procedural coding system (HCPCS). Subsequently, HCFA in 1986 extends the requirement to state medical agencies using the Medicaid Management Information System

1984
AMA provides diagnostic and treatment guidelines for cases involving child abuse and neglect

1985
Judicial Council becomes Council on Ethical and Judicial Affairs

AMA encourages continuing research and studies concerning AIDS

AMA requests adequate government funding for research on AIDS

AMA calls for ban on all tobacco advertising and supports passage of legislation prohibiting smoking on public transportation

1986
AMA passes resolution opposing acts of discrimination against AIDS patients and any legislation that would lead to such categorical discrimination or that would involve patient-physician confidentiality

AMA Board of Trustees establishes the Medical School Visitation Program

AMA establishes the Young Physicians Section

AMA establishes an initiative to improve adolescent health

AMA publicizes and recommends the incorporation of CPR classes in secondary schools

AMA provides professional guidelines relating to a physician's personal, clinical, and public conduct relating to AIDS

AMA adopts policy prohibiting investment of AMA funds in tobacco stocks and urging medical schools and parent universities to eliminate investments in corporations that produce or promote use of tobacco

1987
AMA outlines a comprehensive approach for the prevention and control of AIDS and adopts an AIDS public awareness and information program

AMA establishes Department of Adolescent Health

AMA helps initiate the Surgeon General's workshop on Self-care and Public Health

AMA urges physicians to refer women for mammograms

In *School Board of Nassau County v Gene H. Arline,* US Supreme Court rules that individuals with infectious diseases are considered "handicapped" under anti-discrimination laws, protecting their employment under certain circumstances, as outlined in a friend-of-the-court brief provided by the AMA

AMA urges residency programs to revise requirements to reduce stress and fatigue caused by long hours and to increase supervision of residents

The Joint Commission on the Accreditation of Hospitals becomes the Joint Commission on the Accreditation of Healthcare Organizations

1988
AMA launches the Chinese edition of *Archives of Ophthalmology,* the first of 19 international editions of AMA specialty journals established between 1988 and 1996

AMA publishes and disseminates 420,000 copies of *HIV Blood Test Counseling: AMA Physician Guidelines*

AMA establishes Office of HIV/AIDS

AMA establishes Department of Geriatric Health

AMA works with the Educational Commission for Foreign Medical Graduates to establish the International Medical Scholars Program, to assist foreign physicians to gain access to educational opportunities in the United States

1989

AMA develops National HIV Policy reiterating physicians' ethical responsibility to treat HIV patients whose condition is within the physicians' realm of competence

AMA recommends confidential HIV testing be readily available to all who wish to be tested

AMA establishes the JAMA Journal Club, as a means of earning credit toward the Physician's Recognition Award for continuing education completed

AMA files brief on behalf of Cruzan family in US Supreme Court case *Cruzan v Missouri Department of Health;* AMA holds that the guardian has a right to refuse medical treatment for a patient in a persistent vegetative state. Court later rules that states have the right to regulate food withdrawal

AMA Encyclopedia of Medicine is published by Random House

1990

AMA moves into new building at 515 N State St, Chicago, Ill

AMA publishes *America's Adolescents: How Healthy Are They?*

AMA publishes *HIV Early Care: AMA Physician Guidelines* and disseminates to 350,000 physicians

AMA launches corporate identity program

AMA adopts guidelines governing gifts to physicians from industry

AMA Fellowship Residency Electronic Interactive Data Access System (FREIDA) describing residency programs in the United States is available in electronic form

1991

AMA proposes reform of the US health care system (Health Access America) to include expansion of health insurance coverage

AMA launches campaign against family violence

1992

Archives of Family Medicine founded

AMA calls on tobacco companies to refrain from engaging in advertising practices that target children

AMA adopts a recommendation from the Council on Medical Education that continued federal funding should be available for graduate medical education

AMA Council on Medical Education and Council on Medical Service submit a joint report to House of Delegates identifying major barriers to adequate health care for the inner-city poor and present recommendations for addressing the problems

1993

AMA Auxiliary becomes Alliance

AMA passes resolution declaring physician-assisted suicide is fundamentally inconsistent with the physician's professional role

AMA Council on Medical Education recommends multifaceted approach to encourage student and physician interest in primary care

1994

American Journal of Diseases of Children becomes *Archives of Pediatrics and Adolescent Medicine*

AMA drafts the Patient Protection Act, elements of which were included in every health system reform bill reported out of committee in both the House and Senate

AMA Physician's Recognition Award for completing continuing education is extended to appropriately licensed physicians in Mexico

Commission on Accreditation of Allied Health Education Programs succeeds AMA Committee on Allied Health Education and Accreditation

AMA Council on Medical Education and Council on Long Range Planning and Development submit report analyzing physician work-force planning strategies in light of the impact of health system reform on medical education and academic medical centers

1995

AMA launches grassroots campaign for professional liability reform

AMA drafts the Patient Protection Act II bill with two goals: protection for patients through increased disclosure requirement and managed care fairness; and physicians' need to have defined rights and protections from arbitrary separation from managed care plans

AMA launches its Website on the Internet, featuring highlights of *JAMA,* the specialty journals, *American Medical News,* and other AMA news of interest

JAMA publishes historic issue with six articles examining tobacco industry through corporate documents of Brown and Williamson Tobacco Company

1996

AMA Fellowship Residency Electronic Interactive Data Access System (FREIDA) describing residency programs in the United States goes on-line

On-Line CME Locator is launched by the AMA, featuring more than 2000 Category 1 activities sponsored by accredited providers

AMA, with the American College of Physicians and American College of Surgeons, begins campaign to promote organ and tissue donation for transplantation

AMA House of Delegates gives a voting seat to three organizations with longtime observer status in the House: National Medical Association, American Medical Women's Association, and the American Osteopathic Association

AMA establishes a section for International Medical Graduates with a voting seat in the House

1997

AMA celebrates the sesquicentennial of its founding

AMA launches the American Medical Accreditation Program to reassert the AMA's historic role as the rightful arbiter of physician quality

AMA offers Congress a reform plan to save Medicare for today's seniors and tomorrow's children

AMA establishes the National Patient Safety Foundation to fund research into ways to reduce medical errors and make health care delivery safer

To expand and enhance its role as the voice of professionalism and ethics for the nation's physicians, AMA establishes the Ethics Institute

Index

In this index, page numbers for photographs and illustrations appear in italics. Items listed in the "Highlights in AMA History" timeline (pages 2 through 9) and "A Chronology 1847–1997" (pages 160 through 165) are included in this index.

Photo Credits

Front Matter

p i: Copyright, American Medical Association, 1996.

p ii: Courtesy, National Library of Medicine.

p v: Copyright, American Medical Association, 1996.

p vii: Copyright, American Medical Association, 1996.

p viii: Courtesy, Smithsonian Institution; published with permission of New York City Department of Health.

Timeline

pp 2–3: Background: University Archives, Library of Health Sciences, University of Illinois at Chicago.

p 2: Courtesy, American Medical Association Archives.

p 3: Top left: courtesy of Pennsylvania Hospital, Philadelphia; center: copyright, American Medical Association, 1883.

pp 4–5: Background: Jane Addams Memorial Collection, University Library, University of Illinois at Chicago.

p 4: Center left: courtesy, Temple University; top right: The University of Pennsylvania Archives.

p 5: Courtesy, National Library of Medicine.

pp 6–7: Background: courtesy, Smithsonian Institution; permission to publish by American Lung Association of Western Pennsylvania.

p 6: Center left: courtesy, National Library of Medicine; top right: courtesy, American Medical Association Archives.

p 7: Courtesy, American Medical Association Archives.

pp 8–9: Background: copyright, American Medical Association, 1992.

p 8: Copyright, American Medical Association, 1996; courtesy, Rush-Presbyterian-St Luke's Medical Center, Chicago.

p 9: Top left: *JAMA*, copyright, American Medical Association, 1992; cover artwork, courtesy, Allentown Art Museum, Allentown, Pa; center: copyright, American Medical Association, 1996.

Chapter 1

pp 10–11: Courtesy of Pennsylvania Hospital, Philadelphia.

p 13: Courtesy, American Medical Association Archives.

p 14: The University of Pennsylvania Archives.

p 15: Top: Parke-Davis; bottom: Chicago Historical Society, photograph ICHi-08186.

p 16: Chicago Historical Society, photograph ICHi-22081.

p 17: Courtesy, Museum of the City of New York.

p 19: Courtesy, American Medical Association Archives.

p 20: Copyright, American Medical Association, 1883.

p 21: Library, The Academy of Natural Sciences of Philadelphia.

p 22: Courtesy, National Library of Medicine.

Chapter 2

pp 24–25: Courtesy, Library of Congress, Farm Security Administration Collection.

p 27: Courtesy, American Medical Association Archives.

p 28: Courtesy, National Library of Medicine.

p 29: Courtesy, American Medical Association Archives.

p 30: Copyright, American Medical Association, 1996.

p 31: Courtesy, American Medical Association Archives.

p 32: Courtesy, American Medical Association Archives.

p 33: Courtesy, American Medical Association Archives.

p 35: Copyright, American Medical Association, 1996.

p 37: Top: courtesy, Library of Congress, Farm Security Administration Collection; bottom: courtesy, American Medical Association Archives.

Chapter 3

pp 38–39: Courtesy, Temple University.

p 41: Top: courtesy, American Medical Association Archives; center: courtesy, American Medical Association Archives; bottom: courtesy, American Medical Association Archives.

p 42: Courtesy, National Library of Medicine.

p 43: Center: courtesy, American Medical Association Archives; bottom right: Denver Public Library, Western History Department.

p 44: Top: courtesy, National Library of Medicine; bottom: courtesy, American Medical Association Archives.

p 45: Top: courtesy, American Medical Association Archives; bottom: courtesy, National Library of Medicine.

p 46: Courtesy, American Medical Association Alliance.

p 47: Top: copyright, American Medical Association, 1965; bottom: courtesy, American Medical Association Alliance.

p 48: Courtesy, Smithsonian Institution; published with permission of New York City Department of Health.

p 49: Courtesy, American Medical Association Archives.

p 50: Jane Addams Memorial Collection, University Library, University of Illinois at Chicago.

p 51: Courtesy, Temple University.

p 52: Courtesy, American Medical Association Archives.

p 53: Courtesy, Library of Congress, Name File.

p 54: Courtesy, Library of Congress, Farm Security Administration Collection.

p 55: Courtesy, Smithsonian Institution; published with permission of New York City Department of Health.

Chapter 4

pp 56–57: University Archives, Library of Health Sciences, University of Illinois at Chicago.

p 59: The University of Pennsylvania Archives.

p 60: Courtesy, American Medical Association Archives.

p 61: Northwestern Memorial Hospital Archives.

p 62: Historical Collections, College of Physicians of Philadelphia.

p 63: University Archives, Library of Health Sciences, University of Illinois at Chicago.

p 64: Courtesy, American Medical Association Archives.

p 65: The University of Pennsylvania Archives.

p 66: Courtesy, Rush-Presbyterian-St Luke's Medical Center Archives.

p 67: Copyright, American Medical Association, 1996.

Chapter 5

pp 68–69: Courtesy, National Library of Medicine.

p 71: University Archives, Library of Health Sciences, University of Illinois at Chicago.

p 72: Chicago Historical Society, photograph ICHi-22653.

p 73: Courtesy, National Archives and Records Administration, Signal Corps Record Group.

p 74: Top: courtesy, American Medical Association Archives; bottom: courtesy, American Medical Association Archives.

p 75: Courtesy, American Medical Association Archives.

pp 76–77: Courtesy, American Medical Association Archives.

p 78: Courtesy, American Medical Association Archives.

p 79: Courtesy, American Medical Association Archives.

174

Chapter 6

pp 80–81: State Historical Society of Wisconsin.

p 83: Courtesy, National Library of Medicine.

p 84: Top left: courtesy, NBC/Globe Photos, Inc; top right: copyright, Capital Cities/ABC, Inc, 1996.

p 85: Left: copyright, Capital Cities/ABC, Inc, 1996; right: courtesy, NBC/Globe Photos, Inc.

p 86: Courtesy, American Medical Association Archives.

p 87: Courtesy, American Medical Association Archives.

p 88: Courtesy, American Medical Association Archives.

p 89: Courtesy, National Archives Records Administration, Signal Corps Record Group.

p 90: Courtesy, National Library of Medicine.

p 91: Courtesy, Library of Congress, Name File.

p 92: Courtesy, National Archives and Records Administration/Bettman Archive.

p 93: Courtesy, National Library of Medicine.

Chapter 7

pp 94–95: Courtesy, American Medical Association Archives.

p 97: Courtesy, American Medical Association Archives.

p 98: Courtesy, Library of Congress, Farm Security Administration Collection.

p 99: Copyright, American Medical Association, 1996.

p 100: Courtesy, American Medical Association Archives.

p 101: Copyright, American Medical Association, 1973.

p 103: Courtesy, American Medical Association Archives.

p 105: Top: courtesy, National Aeronautics and Space Administration, Lyndon B. Johnson Space Center, Houston, Tex; bottom: courtesy, National Aeronautics and Space Administration, Lyndon B. Johnson Space Center, Houston, Tex.

Chapter 8

pp 106–107: Courtesy, American Medical Association Archives.

p 109: Background: courtesy, American Medical Association Archives; foreground: courtesy, American Medical Association Archives.

p 110: Top: courtesy, National Library of Medicine; bottom: courtesy, American Medical Association Archives.

p 111: Courtesy, American Medical Association Archives.

p 112: *JAMA,* copyright, American Medical Association, 1977; cover artwork, photograph, copyright, The Art Institute of Chicago, 1996, all rights reserved.

p 113: Left: *JAMA,* copyright, American Medical Association, 1983; cover artwork, courtesy, Maruki Art Museum, Saitama-Ken, Japan; center: *JAMA,* copyright, American Medical Association, 1986; cover artwork, courtesy, National Museum of Vincent van Gogh, Stedelijk Museum, Amsterdam, the Netherlands; right: *JAMA,* copyright, American Medical Association, 1983; cover artwork, courtesy, Jefferson Medical College of Thomas Jefferson University, Philadelphia.

p 114: Left: *JAMA,* copyright, American Medical Association, 1991; cover artwork, courtesy, Terra Museum of American Art, Chicago; top right: *JAMA,* copyright, American Medical Association, 1992; cover artwork, copyright, The Munch Museum, The Munch-Ellingsen Group, ARS, New York, 1992.

p 115: Top right background: copyright, American Medical Association, 1984; top right foreground: *JAMA,* copyright, American Medical Association, 1985; bottom: copyright, American Medical Association, 1996.

p 116: Copyright, Random House, Inc, 1996; courtesy, American Medical Association Archives.

p 117: Copyright, American Medical Association, 1996.

p 119: Copyright, American Medical Association, 1996.

Chapter 9

pp 120–121: Courtesy, National Aeronautics and Space Administration, Lyndon B. Johnson Space Center, Houston, Tex.

p 122: *JAMA,* copyright, American Medical Association, 1986; cover artwork, courtesy, University of California School of Medicine.

p 124: Courtesy, National Library of Medicine/California State University.

p 125: Courtesy, National Library of Medicine/Indiana State Board of Health.

p 126: *JAMA,* copyright, American Medical Association, 1993; cover artwork, courtesy, Brent Jones, photojournalist, Chicago.

p 128: Courtesy, American Medical Association Archives.

p 129: Courtesy, American Medical Association Archives.

p 130: Courtesy, American Medical Association Archives.

p 131: Copyright, American Medical Association, 1996.

Chapter 10

pp 132–133: Courtesy, National Archives and Records Administration, Bettman Archive.

p 135: Copyright, American Medical Association, 1996.

p 136: Courtesy, American Medical Association Archives.

p 137: Left: copyright, American Medical Association, 1996; right: copyright, American Medical Association, 1996.

p 139: Courtesy, American Medical Association Archives.

p 141: Courtesy, American Medical Association Archives.

p 142: Courtesy, American Medical Association Archives.

p 144: Courtesy, American Medical Association Archives.

p 145: Courtesy, American Medical Association Archives.

Chapter 11

pp 146–147: Copyright, American Medical Association, 1996; courtesy, Rush-Presbyterian-St Luke's Medical Center, Chicago.

p 149: Copyright, American Medical Association, 1995.

p 150: Top: copyright, American Medical Association, 1996; center: copyright, American Medical Association, 1996; bottom: copyright, American Medical Association, 1996.

p 151: Top: copyright, American Medical Association, 1996; center: courtesy, American Medical Association Archives; bottom: copyright, American Medical Association, 1992.

p 152: Copyright, American Medical Association, 1992.

p 153: Copyright, American Medical Association, 1992.

pp 154–155: Copyright, American Medical Association, 1996; Panoramic Photography, Cedar Lake, Ind.

p 156: Copyright, American Medical Association, 1996.

p 157: Copyright, American Medical Association, 1996.

p 158: Copyright, American Medical Association, 1996.

p 159: Courtesy, Loyola University Medical Center, Maywood, Ill.